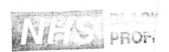

MCQs for the Companion to Psychiatric Studies

Commissioning editor. Michael Parkinson
Project development manager. Barbara Simmons
Project manager. Nancy Arnott
Designer. Erik Bigland

MCQs for the Companion to Psychiatric Studies

Edited by

Stephen M Lawrie MB ChB MRCPsych MPhil MD(Hons)
Senior Clinical Research Fellow,
Department of Psychiatry,
University of Edinburgh,
Royal Edinburgh Hospital, Edinburgh, UK

Michael Sharpe MA MB BChir MRCP MRCPsych
Senior Lecturer in Psychological Medicine,
Department of Psychiatry,
University of Edinburgh,
Royal Edinburgh Hospital, Edinburgh, UK

Eve C Johnstone MD FRCP (Glasgow and Edinburgh) FRCPsych
Professor, Department of Psychiatry,
University of Edinburgh,
Royal Edinburgh Hospital, Edinburgh, UK

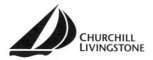

CHURCHILL
LIVINGSTONE

EDINBURGH LONDON NEW YORK PHILADELPHIA ST LOUIS SYDNEY
TORONTO 2000

CHURCHILL LIVINGSTONE
An imprint of Harcourt Publishing Limited

Churchill Livingstone, 1–3 Baxter's Place, Leith Walk,
Edinburgh EH1 3AF

ISBN 0443 064334

British Library of Cataloguing in Publication Data
A catalogue record for this book is available from the
British Library.

**Library of Congress Cataloging in Publication
Data**
A catalog record for this book is available from the
Library of Congress.

Medical knowledge is constantly changing. As
information becomes available, changes in treatment,
procedures, equipment and the use of drugs become
necessary. The author and publisher have, as far as it is
possible, taken care to ensure that the information
given in the text is accurate and up-to-date. However,
readers are strongly advised to confirm that the
information, especially with regard to drug usage,
complies with current legislation and standards of
practice.

The
publisher's
policy is to use
paper manufactured
from sustainable forests

Printed in China

Preface

This book has been designed to accompany the Edinburgh *Companion to Psychiatric Studies*, 6th edition. It is a study aid which uses a multiple choice question format. It is not a revision guide to the MRCPsych, but trainees preparing for the examination are likely to find the MCQ practice and any new approach to learning beneficial. We should stress that the book can be used with or without the *Companion*, but does not replace it.

The book is organised into the same chapters, in the same order, as the *Companion*. The chapters generally contain about 14 questions, each of which follows the standard format of a stem and five questions to be answered true/false. Some chapters, however (e.g. History), do not lend themselves to such an approach and accordingly have had fewer questions taken from them. Each question gives the page number(s) of the *Companion* where the answers can be found. In addition, wherever possible, we give a brief explanation or justification of the true/false answers given. This means that the book can be used as a self-contained study aid and you do not have to carry the rather heavy *Companion* wherever you go. There are, however, some answers without an explanatory note – some 'trues' are bald facts and some 'falses' are just plain wrong.

We are aware that descriptive terms, such as 'commonly', are often imprecise and a source of anxiety for examinees. We have therefore tried to avoid such terms wherever possible. Where it has not been possible to avoid them altogether, we have quoted direct from the *Companion* itself.

We hope that you find the book useful.

Edinburgh 2000

S.M.L.
M.S.
E.C.J.

Contributors

Adam J Burnel MB ChB MRCPsych MPhil
Consultant in General Adult Psychiatry, Murray Royal Hospital,
Perth
11. *Organic disorders*
21. *Personality*
23. *Psychiatric disorders in childhood*

Alan Carson MB ChB MPhil MRCPsych
Lecturer in General Adult and Liaison Psychiatry, University of
Edinburgh, Edinburgh
1. *History of psychiatry*
3. *Neuropharmacology*
4. *Clinical pharmacology*

Jonathan Cavanagh MB ChB MRCPsych MPhil
Research Fellow, University of Edinburgh, Edinburgh
2. *Functional neuroanatomy*
7. *Genetics*
14. *Mood disorder*

Robert A Clafferty MB ChB DGM MRCPsych
Clinical Research Fellow, University of Edinburgh, Edinburgh
17. *Neurotic disorders*
24. *Psychiatric disorders in adolescence*
25. *Old age psychiatry*

John Crichton BmedSci BM BS PhD MRCPsych
Lecturer in Forensic Psychiatry, University of Edinburgh, Edinburgh
12. *Substance misuse*
28. *Forensic psychiatry*
29. *Ethics*

Gillian A Doody BSc MB BS MPhil MRCPsych MD
Lecturer in General Adult Psychiatry, University of Edinburgh, Edinburgh
13. *Schizophrenia*
15. *Paranoid disorders*
16. *Neuroimaging*
22. *Learning disability*

Siobhan MacHale MB BCh BAO MRCPI MRCPsych MPhil
Consultant Liaison Psychiatrist, Royal Edinburgh Hospital, Edinburgh
19. *Sexual disorders*
26. *Suicide*
27. *Liaison psychiatry*

Joanna Smith MA MB ChB
Senior House Officer in Psychiatry, Royal Edinburgh Hospital, Edinburgh
8. *Psychiatric interviewing*
9. *Mental state examination*
10. *Diagnosis*

Robby Steel MA MB ChB MRCPsych
Lecturer in General Adult Psychiatry, University of Edinburgh, Edinburgh
5. *Research methods*
6. *Epidemiology*
31. *Evidence-based medicine*

Deepa Tilak-Singh MB BS MRCPsych
Senior Registrar in General Adult Psychiatry and Psychotherapy, Royal Edinburgh Hospital
18. *Eating disorders*
20. *Women's disorders*
30. *Psychological therapies*

Contents

1. History of psychiatry   1

2. Functional neuroanatomy   5

3. Neuropharmacology   17

4. Clinical pharmacology   29

5. Research methods   41

6. Epidemiology   51

7. Genetics   59

8. Psychiatric interviewing   73

9. Mental state examination   77

10. Diagnosis   85

11. Organic disorders   89

12. Substance misuse   95

13. Schizophrenia   103

14. Mood disorder   111

15. Paranoid disorders   123

16. Neuroimaging   129

17. Neurotic disorders   137

18. Eating disorders   143

19. Sexual disorders   149

20. Women's disorders   155

21. Personality   163

22. Learning disability   171

23. Psychiatric disorders in childhood   179

24. Psychiatric disorders in adolescence   185

25. Old age psychiatry   191

26. Suicide   197

27. Liaison psychiatry   205

28. Forensic psychiatry   215

29. Ethics   223

30. Psychological therapies   231

31. Evidence-based medicine and psychiatry   239

Index   303

1. History of psychiatry

1.1   **Regarding the early history of psychiatry:**

  A   The ancient Greeks described four conditions: phrenitis, mania, melancholia and paranoia.

  B   Lunacy legislation in England dates from the 15th century.

  C   A shift in thinking occurred at the beginning of the Middle Ages and psychiatric conditions began to be thought of as predominantly 'medical'.

  D   Sydenham's textbook (1696) can be regarded as a turning point for modern diagnosis and classification.

  E   The 'madness' of King George III led to a House of Lords enquiry into the treatment of the mentally ill.

1.2   **Regarding the period of humane reform in the treatment of the mentally ill:**

  A   Philippe Pinel is generally credited with popularising treatments involving non-restraint.

  B   William Tuke began 'moral treatment' of the insane at the Retreat in York.

  C   In England, in 1808, a bill was passed for the purpose of providing 'better care and maintenance of lunatics being paupers or criminals'.

  D   The Lunacy Commission was formed in 1845.

  E   The old Lunacy Commission and Board of Control were resurrected in 1983 in the form of the Mental Welfare Commission.

(Answers overleaf)

1.1   **A**   **True**
          B   **False**   Lunacy legislation dates from the 19th century.
          C   **False**   This shift in thinking probably dates to the end of the 18th century.
          D   **True**   It regarded diseases as constellations of symptoms.
          E   **True**

(Further details can be found in the *Companion to Psychiatric Studies*, pp. 1–2.)

1.2   **A**   **True**   He started this work at the Bicetre in 1794.
          B   **True**   The Retreat was opened in 1796.
          C   **True**   The reforms begun by Tuke were followed by the introduction of this bill.
          D   **True**
          E   **True**

(Further details can be found in the *Companion to Psychiatric Studies*, p. 2.)

1.3 **Regarding the development of academic psychiatry:**
A European academic psychiatry began with the publishing of Pinel's *Traité de la Manie.*
B Kraepelin was appointed to the first Chair of Psychiatry and Neurology in Berlin in 1865.
C The first Chair of Psychiatry in Britain was set up in London in 1876.
D German classification schemes developed at the turn of the 20th century have been influential on almost all modern classification systems as they were based on the natural course of mental disorders.
E Bayle's description of 'arachnitis chronique' in 1822 was the first example in psychiatry of a demonstrable pathology in clinical syndromes.

1.4 **The following are correctly associated:**
A Kraepelin – schizophrenia.
B Kahlbaum – developmental insanity.
C Hecker – dementia praecox.
D Bleuler – catatonia.
E Clouston – hebephrenia.

1.5 **Regarding the effects of the First World War:**
A At the beginning of WW1 'shell shock' was viewed analogously to compensation claims after railway accidents.
B Shell shock reached a peak incidence following the Battle of the Somme in 1916.
C Mott considered that there was a pathological basis for shell shock, consisting of minute haemorrhages in the brain.
D From the military perspective the difference between intentional and unintentional symptoms was of the utmost importance.
E Shell shock led to an acceptance among the general public that overwhelming stress could lead to illness even among those of previously proven bravery.

1.6 **The following are correctly associated:**
A Insulin coma therapy – Cade.
B Electroconvulsive treatment – Cerletti and Bini.
C Lithium – Sakel.
D Psychosurgery – Kuhn.
E Imipramine – Moniz.

(Answers overleaf)

1.3   A   **True**   It was published in 1801.
      B   **False**   This was Griesinger's appointment.
      C   **False**   The first Chair of Psychiatry in Britain was set up in Edinburgh in 1919.
      D   **True**
      E   **True**   The disorder was also known as 'general paralysis of the insane'.

(Further details can be found in the *Companion to Psychiatric Studies*, pp. 2–3.)

1.4   A   **False**   The correct association is: Kraepelin – dementia paranoides/dementia praecox/manic-depressive insanity.
      B   **False**   The correct association is: Kahlbaum – catatonia.
      C   **False**   The correct association is: Hecker – hebephrenia.
      D   **False**   The correct association is: Bleuler – schizophrenia.
      E   **False**   The correct association is: Clouston – developmental insanity.

(Further details can be found in the *Companion to Psychiatric Studies*, p. 3.)

1.5   A   **False**
      B   **True**
      C   **True**
      D   **True**
      E   **True**

(Further details can be found in the *Companion to Psychiatric Studies*, pp. 4–5.)

1.6   A   **False**   Sakel introduced insulin coma therapy in 1932.
      B   **True**   Electroconvulsive treatment was introduced by Cerletti and Bini in 1938.
      C   **False**   Cade introduced lithium in 1949.
      D   **False**   Moniz introduced psychosurgery in 1935.
      E   **False**   Kuhn introduced imipramine in 1958.

(Further details can be found in the *Companion to Psychiatric Studies*, p. 5.)

2. Functional neuroanatomy

2.1   **Concerning the cortex and sensory systems:**
A   The cortex consists of six layers.
B   The first cortical layer lies above the pia layer.
C   The final retinal output is from ganglion cells.
D   Retinal ganglion cells have circular receptive fields.
E   The midbrain pretectal area controls pupillary reflexes.

2.2   **Regarding the cerebellum:**
A   It projects to the ventral lateral thalamus via the dentate nucleus.
B   The ventrolateral portion of the dentate nucleus projects to the prefrontal cortex.
C   The main neurotransmitter in granule cells is gamma-aminobutyric acid (GABA).
D   Most cerebellar neurones are excitatory.
E   Purkinje cell output to the dentate nucleus is inhibitory.

2.3   **Basal ganglia structures include:**
A   Nucleus accumbens.
B   Ventral tegmental area.
C   Insula.
D   Diencephalon.
E   Subthalamic nucleus.

(Answers overleaf)

2.1   A   **True**   The cortical sheet is a laminar structure consisting of six layers.

      B   **False**   Layer 1 lies below the pia.

      C   **True**   The axons form the optic nerves.

      D   **True**

      E   **True**

(Further details can be found in the *Companion to Psychiatric Studies*, pp. 15–17.)

2.2   A   **True**   The cerebellum projects via the dentate nucleus to the ventral lateral thalamus and back to areas 4 and 6 thus closing a functional loop allowing the cerebellum to act as motor modulator.

      B   **True**   The ventrolateral portion of dentate may be involved in cognitive processes.

      C   **False**   Granule cells are the only excitatory (glutaminergic) neurones in the cerebellum.

      D   **False**   See above.

      E   **True**   All other cells are inhibitory, using GABA or taurine.

(Further details can be found in the *Companion to Psychiatric Studies*, pp. 21–22.)

2.3   A   **True**

      B   **True**

      C   **False**

      D   **False**

      E   **True**

Basal ganglia structures include the caudate, putamen and ventral striatum (nucleus accumbens); the internal section of the globus pallidus, ventral pallidum, substantia nigra pars reticulata; the globus pallidus external section, subthalamic nucleus, substantia nigra pars compacta and the ventral tegmental area. (Further details can be found in the *Companion to Psychiatric Studies*, p. 22 (Fig. 2.7).)

2.4   **The prefrontal circuit:**
   A   Has been implicated in cognitive function.
   B   Receives input from the substantia nigra.
   C   Receives a direct projection from the posterior association cortex.
   D   Is involved in the control of working memory.
   E   Has links with the basal ganglia.

2.5   **In the frontal 'dementias':**
   A   Apathy is characteristic of dorsolateral prefrontal cortex (DLPFC) atrophy.
   B   The basal ganglia are invariably involved.
   C   Huntington's chorea invariably involves frontal symptoms.
   D   Prefrontal cortex overactivity is present in severe depression.
   E   Hypofrontality in schizophrenia is most frequently reported in the orbitofrontal cortex.

2.6   **The limbic system:**
   A   Is implicated in aspects of memory and emotion.
   B   Has a circuit, described by Papez, encompassing hypothalamus, anterior thalamic nucleus, cingulate cortex and hippocampus.
   C   Incorporates the olfactory bulbs and lobes.
   D   Includes the inferior colliculus.
   E   Includes the globus pallidus.

(Answers overleaf)

2.4   A   **True**   Particularly in working memory.

B   **True**   It receives input from a loop that includes head of caudate, substantia nigra and globus pallidus via ventral anterior and medial dorsal nuclei of the thalamus.

C   **False**   Both posterior parietal association cortex and premotor cortex project into this circuit via the head of caudate.

D   **True**   The most convincing explanation of neuronal function in this area is that it subserves working memory, although this is not fully established.

E   **True**   See B above.

(Further details can be found in the *Companion to Psychiatric Studies*, p. 23.)

2.5   A   **True**   Frontal dementias typically present with overactive disinhibition in orbitofrontal atrophy and apathy in DLPFC atrophy.

B   **True**

C   **False**   Primarily subcortical dementias, e.g. Huntington's, are only occasionally associated with a subcortical dementia of a 'frontal' type.

D   **False**   Severe depression is associated with underactivity of the basal ganglia and prefrontal cortex.

E   **False**   Hypofrontality in schizophrenia is most commonly reported in the DLPFC.

(Further details can be found in the *Companion to Psychiatric Studies*, p. 24.)

2.6   A   **True**
B   **True**
C   **True**
D   **False**
E   **False**

(Further details can be found in the *Companion to Psychiatric Studies*, pp. 24–25.)

2.7   **The hippocampus:**
   A   Has output but no input through the fornix.
   B   Activity is modulated by the locus coeruleus.
   C   Receives a direct projection from the amygdala.
   D   Is known to be involved in memory function, as demonstrated by the neuropathology of Alzheimer's disease.
   E   Is linked to the hypothalamus as part of the original circuit of Papez.

2.8   **Amnesic syndrome:**
   A   Is characterised by anterograde amnesia.
   B   Is associated with clouding of consciousness.
   C   Is accompanied by intact language and intellectual function.
   D   Caused by herpes simplex encephalitis is associated with necrosis of medial temporal structures.
   E   Has prompted studies of brain damage leading to human amnesia which provide key evidence for the involvement of the hippocampus in the biology of memory.

2.9   **The following statements about hippocampal pathology are true:**
   A   The Wernicke–Korsakoff syndrome affects diencephalic structures.
   B   Herpes simplex encephalitis can result in Klüver–Bucy syndrome.
   C   Klüver–Bucy syndrome results from diencephalic damage.
   D   Korsakoff patients can show deficits on frontal lobe testing.
   E   Morphological studies implicate the structure in schizophrenia.

(Answers overleaf)

2.7 A **False** It has both output and input.
  B **True** The locus coeruleus is part of the central noradrenergic system.
  C **True** The hippocampus receives projections from the lateral and basal nuclei of the amygdala.
  D **False** Better evidence of its involvement in memory comes from the amnesic syndrome.
  E **True**

(Further details can be found in the *Companion to Psychiatric Studies*, p. 28.)

2.8 A **True** Amnesic syndrome is characterised by anterograde memory impairment of varying severity usually accompanied by a variable degree of retrograde amnesia in the setting of a clear sensorium with preserved intellectual and language function.
  B **False** See above.
  C **True**
  D **True** Herpes simplex can cause an acute necrotising encephalitis of medial temporal lobes.
  E **False** Uncontrolled illness, varying presentations and deficits additional to core damage hamper the elucidation of the biology of memory.

(Further details can be found in the *Companion to Psychiatric Studies*, p. 28.)

2.9 A **True** Neuropathological examinations of patients with Wernicke–Korsakoff syndrome consistently reveal damage to diencephalic structures, especially the dorsomedial nucleus of the thalamus and mamillary bodies, rather than temporal lobe structures.
  B **True**
  C **False** This results from damage to the anterior temporal lobe, including the amygdala – see *Companion to Psychiatric Studies*, page 32.
  D **True**
  E **True**

(Further details can be found in the *Companion to Psychiatric Studies*, pp. 30–31.)

2.10   Concerning hippocampal morphology in schizophrenia:

A   A reduction in the anterior hippocampus has been
demonstrated using magnetic resonance imaging (MRI).

B   The orientation of hippocampal pyramidal cells is abnormal.

C   Abnormalities on structural imaging give clear evidence of the
genetic basis.

D   The amygdala is usually normal.

E   Some neuropsychological abnormalities in schizophrenia may
be explained by hippocampal abnormalities.

2.11   The hypothalamus:

A   Is linked to the pituitary by the infundibulum.

B   Is divided into medial and lateral nuclei by the fornix.

C   Contains the medial forebrain bundle in the medial region.

D   Contains the supraoptic and paraventricular nuclei in the
posterior portion of the medial region.

E   Contains the nuclei responsible for the secretion of
vasopressin.

2.12   Concerning the function of the amygdala:

A   There is some evidence implicating the amygdala in reactions
to reward stimuli.

B   Electrical stimulation of areas such as the nucleus accumbens
is innately aversive.

C   The amygdaloid complex has been implicated in memory
function.

D   Lesions of the amygdala impair cross-modal memory tasks.

E   Recent studies using positron-emission tomography (PET) in
humans implicate the amygdala in social response.

2.13   Concerning dopaminergic neurones:

A   They are found in the olfactory bulb and the retina.

B   Cell bodies of the 'intermediate' projection systems lie in the
diencephalon.

C   Intermediate cells do not project into the pituitary.

D   The 'long' dopaminergic tracts include the mesolimbic
pathway.

E   The nigrostriatal tract carries fibres from the ultrashort
projection system.

(Answers overleaf)

2.10 **A** **True** MRI studies show significant reductions in medial temporal lobe grey matter, most pronounced in the amygdala and anterior hippocampus.

B **False** Pyramidal cell number and orientation may be abnormal in the hippocampus of some schizophrenics.

C **False** These findings support a neurodevelopmental pathology in schizophrenia.

D **False** See A above.

E **True**

(Further details can be found in the *Companion to Psychiatric Studies*, p. 31.)

2.11 **A** **True**
B **True**
C **False** This is in the lateral region.
D **False** These nuclei are in the anterior portion.
E **True** The supraoptic nuclei produce vasopressin.

(Further details can be found in the *Companion to Psychiatric Studies*, p. 31.)

2.12 **A** **True** This may relate to the neural substrates of affective disorders.

B **False** Electrical stimulation of the nucleus accumbens and related areas is innately rewarding.

C **True**
D **True**
E **True** Recent PET studies in humans have indicated that neural responses in the amygdala may be modulated by photographs showing varied intensities of emotional facial expressions such as happiness and fearfulness.

(Further details can be found in the *Companion to Psychiatric Studies*, p. 33.)

2.13 **A** **True** They form 'ultrashort' projection systems.
B **True**
C **False**
D **True** The three 'long' dopaminergic tracts are the nigrostriatal, mesolimbic and mesocortical.
E **False** The nigrostriatal tract is a long tract.

(Further details can be found in the *Companion to Psychiatric Studies*, p. 34.)

2.14   **Dopaminergic projections:**
   A   Reach the nucleus accumbens.
   B   Do not reach the hippocampus.
   C   From the ventral tegmental area to the nucleus accumbens are implicated in schizophrenia.
   D   In the mesocortical system have been implicated in the pathology of affective disorder.
   E   With differing responses to antipsychotic drugs may explain variations in the side-effect profiles of different drugs.

2.15   **The following statements about the anatomy of the noradrenergic system are true:**
   A   The locus coeruleus contains half the central noradrenergic neurones.
   B   The dorsal noradrenergic bundle projects only to midbrain, thalamus and limbic system.
   C   The ventral noradrenergic bundle innervates the brainstem.
   D   Tegmental noradrenergic neurones provide the principal noradrenergic innervation to the spinal cord.
   E   Locus coeruleus neurones do not have a role in the detection of aversive sensory input.

2.16   **Regarding the anatomy of the serotonergic system:**
   A   The cell bodies of the serotonergic system are the most extensive monoaminergic system.
   B   5-hydroxytryptamine (5-HT) projections to the spinal cord modulate sensory neurones only.
   C   There are no serotonergic projections to the cerebellum.
   D   Serotonergic cell groups project to the locus coeruleus.
   E   The raphe nuclei are located in the midbrain and pons.

(Answers overleaf)

2.14   **A**   **True**   Dopaminergic limbic projections include the nucleus accumbens, the central nucleus of amygdala and the hippocampus.

       B   **False**   See above.

       C   **False**   Frontal activation abnormalities in schizophrenia may be partly mediated by dysfunction in the mesocortical dopamine system, while projections from the ventral tegmental area to the nucleus accumbens – which is increasingly implicated in rewarded behaviour – may play an important role in affective disorder.

       D   **False**   See above.

       E   **True**

(Further details can be found in the *Companion to Psychiatric Studies*, pp. 34–35.)

2.15   **A**   **True**

       B   **False**   They also branch diffusely throughout the cortex.

       C   **True**   It also innervates the hypothalamus and some limbic cortical targets.

       D   **True**

       E   **False**

(Further details can be found in the *Companion to Psychiatric Studies*, p. 35.)

2.16   **A**   **True**

       B   **False**   They also modulate motor neurones.

       C   **False**   There is a small projection to the cerebellum.

       D   **True**

       E   **True**

(Further details can be found in the *Companion to Psychiatric Studies*, pp. 35–36.)

2.17   **Concerning the functional anatomy of the serotonergic system:**
   A   Raphe nuclei project to the cerebral cortex.
   B   Dorsal raphe nuclei project to the nucleus accumbens and frontal cortex.
   C   Median raphe nuclei project to the amygdala.
   D   Raphe nuclei may have a role in mediating responses to acute and chronic aversive events.
   E   Median raphe nuclei have been implicated in the modulation of avoidance behaviour.

2.18   **The following statements concerning the function of the cholinergic system are true:**
   A   The pathology of Alzheimer's disease includes degeneration of the nucleus basalis.
   B   Alzheimer's disease is associated with decreased concentrations of acetylcholinesterase.
   C   Alzheimer's disease is associated with increased concentration of acetylcholine.
   D   Cholinergic changes are the sole monoamine changes found in Alzheimer's disease.
   E   Basalis–amygdala projections may be involved in affective learning.

(Answers overleaf)

2.17 **A** **True** The dorsal and median raphe nuclei have ascending projections to the striatum, limbic system and cortex.
   B **True** The dorsal raphe nucleus (DRN) has projections to the basal ganglia, nucleus accumbens, amygdala and frontal cortex.
   C **False** The median raphe nucleus (MRN) has projection targets in the thalamus, anterior temporal neocortex and hippocampus.
   D **True** It has been proposed that DRN neurones modulate forebrain circuits concerned with evaluative and motor aspects of avoidance behaviour while MRN neurones modulate sensory and memory processing of aversive events.
   E **False** See D above.

(Further details can be found in the *Companion to Psychiatric Studies*, pp. 35–36.)

2.18 **A** **True** The pathology of Alzheimer's disease suggests a particular degeneration of nucleus basalis.
   B **False** Postmortem studies of the brain in Alzheimer's sufferers show reductions in the concentration of acetylcholine and choline acetyltransferase.
   C **False** See B above.
   D **False** The cholinergic system is not the only monoamine system affected in Alzheimer's disease.
   E **True**

(Further details can be found in the *Companion to Psychiatric Studies*, p. 36.)

3. Neuropharmacology

3.1 **Regarding energy and the brain:**
 A The primary energy source is glycogen.
 B The brain accounts for approximately 10% of the body's energy expenditure.
 C Fructose can pass through the blood–brain barrier unimpeded.
 D Under normal circumstances the respiratory quotient (RQ) for the adult brain is 0.71.
 E Nervous tissue contains all the enzymes and metabolic intermediates of anaerobic and aerobic carbohydrate metabolism.

3.2 **According to the rules of pharmacokinetics:**
 A The effective concentration of any drug in relevant tissues depends upon absorption, distribution and excretion but not biotransformation
 B High molecular weight substances cross cell membranes predominantly by passive filtration through aqueous channels.
 C The extent to which a drug is ionised is determined by the pH of its solution and the dissociation constant of the drug.
 D 'Free' drugs pass from plasma to the extracellular fluid of the nervous system at a rate proportional to their concentration gradient.
 E The unionised portion of a drug is more soluble in the lipid bilayer of the cell membrane.

3.3 **Common problems associated with different routes of drug administration include:**
 A Oral: immediate adverse reactions.
 B Subcutaneous: pain and local necrosis.
 C Intramuscular: contraindicated during anticoagulant therapy.
 D Intravenous: unsuitable for oily preparations.
 E Oral: low availability for drugs with high hepatic clearance.

(Answers overleaf)

3.1   A   **False**   The primary source is glucose.
         B   **True**
         C   **False**   Entry into the brain is restricted.
         D   **False**   The brain's RQ is usually 0.99.
         E   **True**   The dependence on glucose is due to impaired substrate transfer across the blood–brain barrier.

(Further details can be found in the *Companion to Psychiatric Studies*, pp. 40–41.)

3.2   A   **False**   Biotransformation is also important.
         B   **False**   Low molecular weight substances, i.e. < 200 Da, move across membranes by passive filtration.
         C   **True**   This is because many drugs are organic electrolytes and weak acids/bases.
         D   **True**
         E   **True**   The unionised portion of a drug is 10 000 times more soluble than the ionised portion.

(Further details can be found in the *Companion to Psychiatric Studies*, p. 43.)

3.3   A   **False**   Such reactions are associated with intravenous administration.
         B   **True**
         C   **True**
         D   **True**
         E   **True**

(Further details can be found in the *Companion to Psychiatric Studies*, p. 44 (Table 3.1).)

3.4   **Regarding the blood–brain barrier:**

A   It is represented functionally by the capillary endothelium of the brain.

B   It allows the pH of the cerebrospinal fluid to be lower than plasma pH.

C   Phenylalanine competes with tryptophan for the same transport system across it.

D   Active transport mechanisms act across it in both directions.

E   Permeability of a the cell membranes to a drug is proportional to the drug's partition coefficient.

3.5   **Regarding biotransformation:**

A   Biotransformation of most drugs takes place in hepatic microsomal enzyme systems.

B   Individual variation can be related to both genetic and environmental factors.

C   The process of biotransformation can lead to activation or inactivation of a drug.

D   Lipid-soluble drugs are more readily excreted.

E   Age has little effect on the process of biotransformation.

3.6   **The following are true of drug clearance:**

A   For most drugs in psychiatry, clearance mechanisms are not saturated during routine clinical usage.

B   Steady states are reached when the rate of drug administration is slightly greater than elimination.

C   When clearance systems for a drug are saturated, its pharmacokinetics become first order.

D   Imipramine is mostly cleared by the kidney.

E   Renal clearance is substantially influenced by protein binding.

3.7   **The following types and examples of substances active in neuronal signalling are correctly paired:**

A   Neurotransmitter – acetylcholine.

B   Neurohormone – steroids.

C   Neuromodulator – nerve growth factor.

D   Neuromediator – cyclic adenosine monophosphate.

E   Neurotrophin – corticotrophin-releasing factor.

(Answers overleaf)

3.4   A   **False**   Capillary endothelium is the structure of the
                        blood–brain barrier.
        B   **True**   It is typically 0.1 pH unit lower.
        C   **True**   As also do valine, leucine and isoleucine.
        D   **True**
        E   **True**   This is the 'pH partition hypothesis'.

(Further details can be found in the *Companion to Psychiatric Studies*, pp. 44–45.)

3.5   A   **True**
        B   **True**
        C   **True**
        D   **False**   They first need to be metabolised into more polar
                        compounds.
        E   **False**   Age exerts a considerable effect.

(Further details can be found in the *Companion to Psychiatric Studies*, pp. 45–46.)

3.6   A   **True**
        B   **False**   Steady state is reached when administration and
                        elimination rates are equal.
        C   **False**   They become zero order, i.e. a constant amount is
                        cleared per unit of time.
        D   **False**   Imipramine is mostly cleared by the liver, lithium by
                        the kidney.
        E   **True**   A drug bound to blood proteins is not filtered.

(Further details can be found in the *Companion to Psychiatric Studies*, p. 46.)

3.7   A   **True**
        B   **False**   Corticotrophin-releasing factor is a neurohormone;
                        steroids are neuromodulators.
        C   **False**
        D   **True**
        E   **False**   Neurotrophin is a nerve growth factor.

(Further details can be found in the *Companion to Psychiatric Studies*, p. 48 (Table 3.3).)

3.8   When a drug binds to a receptor:

A   Certain drugs bind by van der Waals binding.

B   Those that bind to receptors and initiate a response in neuroeffector tissue are agonists.

C   Antagonists have no intrinsic pharmacological activity.

D   Partial agonists can only bind by hydrophobic binding.

E   Drugs that combine both antagonist and agonist properties have no clinical potential.

3.9   With regard to different receptor mechanisms:

A   Thyroid hormone activates the α subunit of its receptor causing it to open wider following the passage of cations.

B   The nicotinic acetylcholine receptor is an example of a ligand-gated ion channel.

C   Steroid hormone receptors consist of a ligand-binding domain and a structural complex that couples the receptor to intracellular metabolic processes.

D   Nerve growth factor acts at a tyrosine kinase-linked receptor.

E   The postsynaptic glycine receptor is a large membrane-spanning glycoprotein complex which when activated forms an anion channel.

3.10   Regarding the GABA receptor:

A   GABA is the main cortical inhibitory neurotransmitter.

B   The $GABA_A$ channel's inhibitory action is chloride dependent.

C   The $GABA_A$ complex has a specific site for the binding of benzodiazepines.

D   Baclofen only binds at $GABA_A$ receptors.

E $GABA_B$ receptors are more widely distributed than $GABA_A$ receptors.

3.11   Regarding excitatory amino acids and their receptors:

A   Excitatory amino acid neurotransmitters are essential in learning and memory.

B   Homocysteic acid is the most abundant excitatory neurotransmitter.

C   Non-NDMA (N-methyl-D-aspartate) receptors are highly concentrated in the cerebellum.

D   Ketamine is a selective agonist at NMDA receptors.

E   Glutamate is a potent neurotoxin.

(Answers overleaf)

3.8 A True
     B True
     C True Antagonists prevent agonists initiating a response.
     D False
     E False Such an opiate could provide analgesia without addiction.

(Further details can be found in the *Companion to Psychiatric Studies*, p. 50.)

3.9 A False Thyroid hormone reduces the inhibitory effects of the receptor structure.
     B True Glutamate and GABA receptors are also examples.
     C True This is also true of thyroid hormone.
     D True
     E True

(Further details can be found in the *Companion to Psychiatric Studies*, pp. 54–55.)

3.10 A True
      B True It is a ligand-gated ion channel.
      C True
      D False Baclofen only binds at $GABA_B$ receptors.
      E False

(Further details can be found in the *Companion to Psychiatric Studies*, pp. 55–57.)

3.11 A True
      B False Glutamate and aspartate are the most abundant.
      C True
      D False Ketamine is a non-competitive antagonist at NMDA receptors.
      E True The phenomenon is termed excitotoxicity.

(Further details can be found in the *Companion to Psychiatric Studies*, pp. 58–59.)

3.12   In cholinergic transmission:
A   Atropine is an antagonist at the 'nicotinic' acetylcholine receptor.
B   'Muscarinic' receptors are G protein-coupled.
C   In vivo, neurones are capable of differential expression of 'nicotinic' receptor subunits.
D   The synthesis of acetylcholine is in a single step catalysed by choline acetyltransferase.
E   Black widow spider venom produces a rapid release of acetylcholine.

3.13   The following are antagonists at nicotinic receptors:
A   Nicotine.
B   Scopolamine.
C   Tubocurarine.
D   Dimethyl-phenylpiperazinium (DMPP).
E   Pilocarpine.

3.14   With regard to anticholinesterase drugs:
A   Anticholinesterases increase presynaptic production of acetylcholine.
B   They were investigated for use in chemical warfare.
C   They act by inhibiting the action of choline acetyltransferase.
D   Physostigmine does not reverse the anticholinergic cardiotoxic effects of tricyclic drugs.
E   Reversible anticholinesterases bind to the enzyme and are oxidised slowly.

3.15   Noradrenergic transmission:
A   At α receptors leads to contraction of the radial muscle of the iris.
B   At β_1 receptors causes bronchodilatation.
C   At α_2 receptors decreases neuronal noradrenaline release.
D   At β_1 receptors increases the rate but not the force of cardiac contractions.
E   At α_1 receptors causes vascular smooth muscle to relax.

3.16   The following are noradrenergic agonists:
A   Prazosin.
B   Clonidine.
C   Salbutamol.
D   Phenylephrine.
E   Yohimbine.

(Answers overleaf)

3.12   A   False   Atropine is a muscarinic antagonist.
       B   True
       C   True   There are multiple forms of two of the four subunits.
       D   True   Acetyl coenzyme A and choline are combined.
       E   True

(Further details can be found in the *Companion to Psychiatric Studies*, pp. 59–60.)

3.13   A   False   Nicotine is an agonist.
       B   False   Scopolamine is a muscarinic antagonist.
       C   True
       D   False   DMPP is an agonist.
       E   False   Pilocarpine is a muscarinic agonist.

(Further details can be found in the *Companion to Psychiatric Studies*, p. 61.)

3.14   A   False   They cause accumulation at synapses.
       B   True
       C   False   They inhibit acetylcholinesterase.
       D   True
       E   False   They are hydrolysed slowly.

(Further details can be found in the *Companion to Psychiatric Studies*, p. 61.)

3.15   A   True   They thus produce pupil dilatation.
       B   False   This is a β_2 effect.
       C   True
       D   False   Both rate and force are increased.
       E   False   They cause contraction of vascular smooth muscle.

(Further details can be found in the *Companion to Psychiatric Studies*, pp. 62–63.)

3.16   A   False   Prazosin is an α_1 antagonist.
       B   True
       C   True
       D   True
       E   False   Yohimbine is an α_2 antagonist.

(Further details can be found in the *Companion to Psychiatric Studies*, p. 63 (Table 3.10).)

3.17   Noradrenaline:

A   Is synthesised by the hydroxylation of dopamine.

B   Is mainly stored in presynaptic complexes with ATP, metallic ions and chromogranins.

C   Reuptake is enhanced by reserpine.

D   Is released from storage vesicles by a potassium-dependent process.

E   Release from storage is inhibited by some antihypertensive agents.

3.18   Regarding the reuptake and degradation of noradrenaline from the synaptic cleft:

A   Reuptake occurs by passive diffusion.

B   Reuptake is affected more by imipramine than desipramine.

C   Cocaine inhibits the presynaptic reuptake.

D   Degradation is predominantly effected by monoamine oxidase type B.

E   Catechol-O-methyl-transferase acts in the degradation process.

3.19   Dopamine:

A   Is synthesised from the hydroxylation of L-dopa.

B   Is released from central dopaminergic terminals by a single mechanism.

C   Release is inhibited by amphetamines.

D   Receptors have at least four subtypes.

E D_1 receptors are the most abundant in the substantia nigra.

3.20   In Parkinson's disease:

A   Cells in the pars compacta of the substantia nigra degenerate.

B   Monoamine oxidase inhibitor type A can slow the progression of symptoms.

C   Surgical treatment aims to reduce activity in indirect D_2 pathways to the substantia nigra.

D   There is a relative deficiency of cholinergic activity.

E   Dopamine agonists are often used as adjuncts to L-dopa in treatment.

(Answers overleaf)

3.17   A   **True**   The enzyme is dopamine β-hydroxylase.
          B   **True**
          C   **False**   Reserpine disrupts storage, which can produce stimulation initially.
          D   **False**   Release is calcium dependent.
          E   **True**   Guanethidine is an example.

(Further details can be found in the *Companion to Psychiatric Studies*, p. 62.)

3.18   A   **False**   Reuptake is energy consuming.
          B   **False**   Secondary amines like desipramine affect noradrenaline more than tertiary amines like imipramine.
          C   **True**
          D   **False**   MAO type A is more effective in degrading noradrenaline, serotonin and dopamine.
          E   **True**

(Further details can be found in the *Companion to Psychiatric Studies*, pp. 64–66.)

3.19   A   **False**   L-tyrosine is hydroxylated to L-dopa, which is decarboxylated to dopamine.
          B   **False**   There are energy- and calcium-dependent release mechanisms.
          C   **False**   Amphetamine facilitates release.
          D   **True**
          E   **False**   They are most abundant in the caudate, nucleus accumbens and olfactory tubercle.

(Further details can be found in the *Companion to Psychiatric Studies*, pp. 66–68.)

3.20   A   **True**
          B   **False**   MAO type B inhibitors can, however.
          C   **True**
          D   **False**   There is a relative excess.
          E   **True**   Bromocriptine is an example.

(Further details can be found in the *Companion to Psychiatric Studies*, pp. 70–71.)

3.21   The following are true of serotonin receptors:

A   Buspirone is an antagonist at $5\text{-}HT_{1A}$ receptors.
B   LSD is a serotonin agonist.
C   ECT increases the number of $5\text{-}HT_2$ receptors.
D   Imipramine reduces the number of $5\text{-}HT_1$ receptors.
E   Ritanserin is a 5-HT agonist.

3.22   Concerning drugs that inhibit serotonin reuptake:

A   Paroxetine is the most potent inhibitor of serotonin reuptake.
B   The clomipramine metabolite desmethyl-clomipramine is also a selective serotonin reuptake inhibitor.
C   A major advantage of fluoxetine is the short half-life of its metabolites.
D   Zimelidine is a good choice in patients with liver failure.
E   Sertraline's clinical actions are greatly enhanced by its active metabolites.

3.23   The following are regarded as evidence of the importance of neural regulation of the endocrine system to psychiatry:

A   The neurotransmitter systems affected by psychiatric drugs are involved in limbic hypothalamic integration and regulation of the pituitary gland.
B   The experimental evidence that hypothalamic releasing factors also function as neurotransmitters.
C   The presence of psychological symptoms in the endocrinopathies.
D   The co-localisation of releasing factors and 'classical neurotransmitters' in the same nerve terminal.
E   Clinical studies implicating stressful stimuli in the pathogenesis of mental illnesses.

3.24   Regarding substances active at opioid receptors:

A   The enkephalins are derived from pro-opiomelanocortin (POMC).
B   Opioid agonist drugs act predominantly at the κ receptor.
C   There is extensive cross-tolerance between opioid drugs.
D   Methadone is chemically distinct from other opioid agonists such as morphine.
E   Opioid dependence and withdrawal may be due to the proliferation of new receptors and their altered sensitivity.

(Answers overleaf)

3.21   A   **False**   It is a selective partial agonist.
        B   **True**   It is a partial 5-HT$_2$ agonist.
        C   **True**
        D   **True**
        E   **False**   It is an antagonist.

(Further details can be found in the *Companion to Psychiatric Studies*, pp. 72–73.)

3.22   A   **True**
        B   **False**   It only inhibits reuptake of noradrenaline.
        C   **False**   The active metabolite norfluoxetine has a half-life of 7–15 days.
        D   **False**   It was withdrawn owing to hepatotoxicity.
        E   **False**   Sertraline metabolites are considerably less active.

(Further details can be found in the *Companion to Psychiatric Studies*, p. 73.)

3.23   A   **True**
        B   **True**
        C   **True**
        D   **True**
        E   **True**

(Further details can be found in the *Companion to Psychiatric Studies*, pp. 74–75.)

3.24   A   **False**   β-endorphin is derived from POMC.
        B   **False**   They act at the μ receptor.
        C   **True**
        D   **True**
        E   **True**

(Further details can be found in the *Companion to Psychiatric Studies*, p. 77.)

4. Clinical psychopharmacology

4.1   Important events in the history of psychopharmacology include:

A   In 1912 John Cade published the first account of the mood-stabilising effects of lithium salts.

B   Paul Charpentier's synthesis of chlorpromazine.

C   The development of monoamine oxidase inhibitors following the observation of the mood-elevating effects of certain antituberculous drugs.

D   The description of imipramine's efficacy in 'vital depression' by Kuhn.

E   The synthesis of clozapine in the early 1980s.

4.2   In general, the following rules apply to the different structural subtypes of antipsychotics:

A   Aliphatic compounds are of high potency.

B   Piperazine compounds have a greater propensity for neurological adverse effects.

C   The butyrophenones are among the most selective D_2 antagonists.

D   The short half-life of the diphenylbutylpiperidines makes them particularly useful for emergency situations.

E   The substituted benzamides are associated with lower rates of extrapyramidal dysfunction.

4.3   The following are believed to be important in explaining the mode of action of antipsychotic drugs:

A   All currently known compounds of proven efficacy block central D_2 receptors at postsynaptic sites.

B D_1 receptors stimulate the synthesis of adenylate cyclase.

C   The D_2 receptor exists as a single isomorph.

D   Clozapine combines D_2 antagonism with marked 5-HT_{2A} antagonism.

E   The dopamine hypothesis of schizophrenia postulates dopamine overactivity in the ventral-tegmental area.

(Answers overleaf)   **29**

4.1	A	**False**	Cade published his account of lithium in 1949.
	B	**True**	Charpentier synthesised chlorpromazine in 1950.
	C	**True**	Monoamine oxidase inhibitors were introduced in 1957.
	D	**True**	Kuhn demonstrated the efficacy of imipramine in 'vital depression' in 1957.
	E	**False**	Clozapine was synthesised in 1958.

(Further details can be found in the *Companion to Psychiatric Studies*, pp. 81–82.)

4.2	A	**False**	Aliphatics tend to be of low potency.
	B	**True**	This is because of their high potency.
	C	**True**	
	D	**False**	They have a long half-life.
	E	**True**	

(Further details can be found in the *Companion to Psychiatric Studies*, pp. 82–84.)

4.3	A	**True**	
	B	**True**	
	C	**False**	D_3 and D_4 isomorphs are part of the D_2 receptor family.
	D	**True**	
	E	**False**	Overactivity is considered to be in the mesolimbic dopaminergic pathway.

(Further details can be found in the *Companion to Psychiatric Studies*, pp. 87–88.)

4.4   **The following adverse effects are frequently associated with antipsychotics:**

A   Weight gain.
B   Hypersalivation.
C   Torsade de pointes.
D   Hyperprolactinaemia.
E   Increase in resting heart rate.

4.5   **The following disorders can be caused by phenothiazines:**

A   Marchiafava–Bignami syndrome.
B   Biliary cirrhosis.
C   Cataract.
D   Systemic lupus erythematosus.
E   Alopecia.

4.6   **Regarding extrapyramidal side-effects of neuroleptics:**

A   30% of acute dystonias will occur in the first week of therapy.
B   The tremor of Parkinson's disease occurs infrequently in the drug-related disorder.
C   Clozapine therapy is often limited by akathisia.
D   Tardive dyskinesia is mild and unobtrusive in the majority of cases.
E   The Chinese are at particular risk of tardive dyskinesia.

4.7   **Regarding the pharmacokinetics of the tricyclic drugs:**

A   They are poorly absorbed from the gastrointestinal tract.
B   They are all subjected to heavy first-pass metabolism effects.
C   Alcohol intoxication, in a non-dependent person, impairs metabolism.
D   The kidney is the major route of elimination.
E   They are 90% unbound in plasma.

4.8   **The muscarinic antagonism of tricyclic drugs is believed to be the main cause of the following side-effects:**

A   Sedation.
B   Erectile difficulties.
C   Impairment of memory.
D   Postural hypotension.
E   Premature ejaculation.

(Answers overleaf)

4.4   **A** **True**
      B **False** Dry mouth, due to anticholinergic effects, is typical.
      C **False** This is rare and usually associated with high doses of thioridazine.
      D **True** This is due to blockade of tuberoinfundibular D_2 receptors.
      E **True**

(Further details can be found in the *Companion to Psychiatric Studies*, pp. 89–91.)

4.5   **A** **False**
      B **True** This is very rare, however.
      C **True** The risk is increased three- to fourfold.
      D **True** This is very rare, however.
      E **True** Hair loss is not infrequent but alopecia areata is rare.

(Further details can be found in the *Companion to Psychiatric Studies*, pp. 91–92.)

4.6   **A** **False** 90% come on within 5 days of exposure.
      B **True**
      C **False** Akathisia is less common on clozapine.
      D **True** Only about 10% are severe.
      E **False** Asians, especially Chinese, have a low risk.

(Further details can be found in the *Companion to Psychiatric Studies*, pp. 94–95.)

4.7   **A** **False** They are well absorbed.
      B **True** Only 50–60% of an oral dose reaches the systemic circulation.
      C **True** Metabolism is impaired by competition.
      D **True**
      E **False** They are 90% bound.

(Further details can be found in the *Companion to Psychiatric Studies*, pp. 100–101.)

4.8   **A** **False**
      B **True** There may be poorly sustained erections or priapism.
      C **True**
      D **False** A mild tachycardia is, however, possible.
      E **False**

(Further details can be found in the *Companion to Psychiatric Studies*, p. 103.)

4.9 **Regarding the effects of tricyclics on the heart:**
A   Tricyclics are class I antiarrhythmics.
B   They have little effect on atrioventricular nodal conduction.
C   They can cause QT shortening on ECG traces.
D   Heart block is highly unlikely in patients with a normal ECG pretreatment.
E   Although sparse, available evidence suggests that tricyclics do not have a negative inotropic effect on the left ventricle.

4.10 **Regarding monoamine oxidase inhibitors:**
A   Isocarboxazid is structurally similar to amphetamine.
B   Phenelzine has a short half-life of 2–4 hours.
C   Tranylcypromine has rapid and almost complete hepatic metabolism.
D   Moclobomide's mode of action has been described as a 'suicide effect'.
E   Acetylator status is the major determinant of efficacy.

4.11 **The following adverse effects are commonly described with monoamine oxidase inhibitors (MAOIs):**
A   Lowering of supine blood pressure.
B   Marked ECG changes.
C   Tachycardia.
D   Dry mouth.
E   Constipation.

4.12 **The following should be excluded from the diet of a patient on monoamine oxidase inhibitors:**
A   Caviar.
B   Champagne.
C   Bananas.
D   Mature Stilton.
E   Fresh herring.

(Answers overleaf)

4.9 A **True** They are membrane stabilisers through inhibition of fast sodium channels.

  B **True** Rather, they can delay intraventricular conduction in the His–Purkinje system.

  C **False** They cause QT prolongation.

  D **True** Only 0.7% of the Roose et al 1987 prospective series of 150 such patients developed heart block.

  E **True**

(Further details can be found in the *Companion to Psychiatric Studies*, pp. 104–106.)

4.10 A **False** Tranylcypromine is similar to amphetamine.

  B **True**

  C **True**

  D **False** This applies to the metabolism of monoamine oxidase inhibitors (MAOIs) in which the enzyme produces intermediates that inactivate it by irreversible binding.

  E **False** Acetylation is probably not involved.

(Further details can be found in the *Companion to Psychiatric Studies*, pp. 106–107.)

4.11 A **True** However, the mechanism is uncertain.

  B **False** MAOIs have no direct effects on rhythm, conduction or contractility.

  C **False** A bradycardia is usual.

  D **True** This is probably due to cholinergic/noradrenergic imbalance.

  E **True** See D above.

(Further details can be found in the *Companion to Psychiatric Studies*, pp. 108–109.)

4.12 A **True**

  B **False** Alcohol is generally safe.

  C **False** Banana skins are to be avoided, however.

  D **True**

  E **False** Only pickled herring should be avoided.

(Further details can be found in the *Companion to Psychiatric Studies*, p. 110.)

4.13   **Regarding the pharmacokinetics of new generation antidepressants:**

A   At high doses metabolism of trazodone produces an active anxiogenic metabolite.

B   Paroxetine inhibits its own metabolism.

C   Fluoxetine has an exceptionally long elimination half-life.

D   In the systemic circulation, venlafaxine is almost completely protein bound.

E   Nefadozone is slowly absorbed from the gastrointestinal tract.

4.14   **The following are thought to be true of the mode of action of selective serotonin reuptake inhibitors:**

A   They block reuptake of serotonin relative to noradrenaline into the presynaptic bulb.

B   They have marked affinity for neurotransmitter receptors.

C   Enhancing biogenic amine transmission is a necessary first step.

D   Fluoxetine is the most potent inhibitor of serotonin reuptake.

E   They all also block noradrenaline uptake.

4.15   **The following well-recognised side-effects are correctly matched:**

A   Mianserin – hyponatraemia.

B   Trazadone – blood dyscrasias.

C   Fluoxetine – priapism.

D   Paroxetine – weight loss.

E   Sertraline – acute dystonia.

4.16   **In overdoses of antidepressants:**

A   The absorption of tricyclic drugs is delayed.

B   At high levels, the pharmacokinetics of tricyclics change from zero order to first order.

C   Delayed atrioventricular conduction is the major cardiac risk.

D   Constricted pupils are a diagnostic clue.

E   Acidaemia can lead to major increases in circulating free drug.

(Answers overleaf)

4.13 A **True** It produces *m*-chlorophenylpiperazine (*m*-CPP).
B **True** So also does fluoxetine.
C **True** Its elimination half-life is 7–15 days.
D **False** Protein binding is low compared to other antidepressants at < 30%.
E **False** It is rapidly absorbed.

(Further details can be found in the *Companion to Psychiatric Studies*, pp. 110–112.)

4.14 A **True**
B **False**
C **True**
D **False** Paroxetine is the most potent.
E **True**

(Further details can be found in the *Companion to Psychiatric Studies*, p. 112.)

4.15 A **False** The correct association is: mianserin – blood dyscrasias.
B **False** The correct association is: trazodone – priapism.
C **False** The correct association is: fluoxetine – agitation.
D **False** Paroxetine is the only selective serotonin reuptake inhibitor (SSRI) not to cause weight loss.
E **True**

(Further details can be found in the *Companion to Psychiatric Studies*, pp. 114–115.)

4.16 A **True** Absorption is substantially delayed, probably by anticholinergic effects.
B **False** The change is from first order to zero order, i.e. the amount metabolised is fixed rather than a proportion.
C **False** They delay ventricular conduction time.
D **False** Pupils are dilated.
E **True** Acidaemia is due to central respiratory depression and a fall in pH reducing protein binding.

(Further details can be found in the *Companion to Psychiatric Studies*, pp. 115–116.)

4.17   The following are true of antidepressant withdrawal syndromes:

A   Akathisia is a recognised feature.
B   Cardiac arrhythmias occur.
C   A prevalence of 70% is generally accepted.
D   Flu-like symptoms are typical of withdrawal syndromes with selective serotonin reuptake inhibitors (SSRIs).
E   Monoamine oxidase inhibitor (MAOI) drugs are free of withdrawal effects.

4.18   Common adverse effects of lithium include:

A   Nausea.
B   Metallic taste in mouth.
C   Increased salivation.
D   Interstitial nephropathy.
E   Hyperthyroidism.

4.19   Regarding lithium toxicity:

A   Diarrhoea is the first symptom in 90% of cases.
B   Clinical signs of central nervous system toxicity closely follow changes in lithium blood levels.
C   Toxicity is usually accompanied by the production of small amounts of concentrated urine.
D   Although theoretically advantageous, 'forced' diuresis is of no benefit in the clinical management of toxic patients.
E   If aware of the early signs of toxicity, patients can often prevent it by omitting medication for a day.

4.20   Regarding benzodiazepines:

A   All are weak organic acids.
B   The rate of absorption is the rate-limiting step in the onset of action.
C   They are subject to extensive first-pass metabolism following absorption from the gastrointestinal tract.
D   Absorption from intramuscular sites is unpredictable.
E   Hepatic metabolism often results in active metabolites.

(Answers overleaf)

4.17 A **True**
      B **True**
      C **False**
      D **True** Symptoms are coryza, myalgia and shaking chills.
      E **False** MAOI withdrawal can be dramatic.

(Further details can be found in the *Companion to Psychiatric Studies*, pp. 116–117.)

4.18 A **True** It occurs in most patients and before steady state is established.
      B **False** This is an infrequent effect.
      C **True**
      D **False** Polyuria is common; nephropathy is rare.
      E **False** Hypothyroidism is common; hyperthyroidism is rare.

(Further details can be found in the *Companion to Psychiatric Studies*, pp. 123–125.)

4.19 A **False** Anorexia and vomiting are usually the first signs.
      B **False** Brain penetration and egression are delayed.
      C **False** Large amounts of dilute urine are produced.
      D **False** Forced diuresis is recommended.
      E **True**

(Further details can be found in the *Companion to Psychiatric Studies*, p. 127.)

4.20 A **False** They are all weak organic bases.
      B **True**
      C **True**
      D **True** However, intramuscular lorazepam is generally rapidly absorbed.
      E **True** There are some exceptions, e.g. lorazepam and temazepam.

(Further details can be found in the *Companion to Psychiatric Studies*, p. 133.)

4.21   Regarding the pharmacodynamics of benzodiazepine drugs:

A   The specific benzodiazepine receptor sites were described in the 1950s.

B   Benzodiazepines react principally with $GABA_B$ receptors.

C   Benzodiazepines facilitate GABA-mediated inhibitory effects in the central nervous system by prolonging the duration of opening of GABA receptors.

D   The mechanism by which GABA stimulation opens the chloride channel involves allosteric modulation.

E   The existence of benzodiazepine receptors implies the existence of a similar endogenous ligand.

4.22   Regarding the adverse effects of benzodiazepines:

A   They have a potent type 1_C antiarrhythmic effect.

B   Impaired psychomotor processing is primarily related to sedation.

C   Impairment of short-term memory is predominantly retrograde.

D   Following termination of treatment, sleep electroencephalograms will show rapid eye movement rebound.

E   Symptoms of withdrawal start within 24 hours of the last drug dose.

4.23   Buspirone:

A   Is a $5-HT_{1A}$ antagonist.

B   Has a long half-life, which allows for once-daily dosing regimes.

C   Requires up to 3 weeks, from first dosage, to develop its clinical effects.

D   Has a marked anticonvulsant action.

E   Has been associated with 'extrapyramidal' side-effects.

4.24   Regarding anticholinergic drugs:

A   They have their principal action at the nicotinic anticholinergic receptors.

B   Orphenadrine is associated with problems of toxicity in overdose.

C   Benztropine has been associated with heat stroke.

D   Anticholinergics can exacerbate acute positive psychotic symptoms.

E   As a group, the anticholinergics tend to cause negative cognitions.

(Answers overleaf)

4.21 A **False** They were discovered in 1977.
B **False** Benzodiazepines do not react with $GABA_B$ receptors.
C **False** They increase the number of opened channels.
D **True** Physical distortion of the complex is thought to occur.
E **True**

(Further details can be found in the *Companion to Psychiatric Studies*, p. 134.)

4.22 A **False** They have little or no autonomic actions.
B **False** There is a primary impairment of information processing.
C **False** Memory impairment is almost entirely anterograde.
D **True**
E **False** They generally start 5–7 days after stopping the drugs.

(Further details can be found in the *Companion to Psychiatric Studies*, pp. 135–136.)

4.23 A **False** It is a partial $5\text{-}HT_{1A}$ agonist.
B **False** It has a half-life of only 2–4 hours.
C **True**
D **False** It is proconvulsant.
E **True** It is a weak dopamine antagonist, albeit on autoreceptors.

(Further details can be found in the *Companion to Psychiatric Studies*, p. 137.)

4.24 A **False** They are muscarinic antagonists.
B **True** It can be fatal in doses of only 10 times the therapeutic dose.
C **True**
D **True**
E **False** They are euphorogenic.

(Further details can be found in the *Companion to Psychiatric Studies*, p. 139.)

5. Research methods

5.1 **The following would typically be included in a study protocol:**
A   A statement of the aims of the study.
B   A statement of the anticipated date and place of publication.
C   A review of relevant literature.
D   Details of the study design and methodology.
E   Copies of the patient information sheet and consent form.

5.2 **In the field of study design:**
A   Observational studies can be used to establish the direction of causality.
B   Selection bias leads to non-random samples and misleading results.
C   Cohort studies provide information about 'relative risk'.
D   Case–control studies give information about prevalance and incidence.
E   Sex can be confounding.

5.3 **When designing a study:**
A   Badly chosen inclusion and exclusion criteria may lead to an underestimate of treatment effects.
B   The contribution made by placebo responders to the result can be established by using a crossover design.
C   It is critical to use a reliable and valid method for establishing diagnosis.
D   Patients who withdraw from the study prematurely should be disregarded.
E   Power calculations are used to estimate how many subjects will be required for the study to stand a good chance of showing a statistically significant result.

(Answers overleaf)

5.1	A	True	The aims should be stated clearly and simply.
	B	False	These are unnecessary and unpredictable.
	C	True	Its purpose is to describe the rationale for the study.
	D	True	
	E	True	

(Further details can be found in the *Companion to Psychiatric Studies*, p. 149 (Table 5.1).)

5.2	A	False	They only give clues to causality; they cannot establish the direction.
	B	True	
	C	True	The relative risk is the ratio of illness in the exposed to the unexposed.
	D	False	Case–control studies give clues to aetiology; surveys are required to estimate disease frequency (see also *Companion to Psychiatric Studies*, p. 199).
	E	True	Confounders are variables that are related to both risk factors and illness.

(Further details can be found in the *Companion to Psychiatric Studies*, pp. 150–151.)

5.3	A	True	It may occur, for example, through recruiting treatment-resistant subjects.
	B	True	Placebo response can be quantified in any controlled study.
	C	True	It reduces sample heterogeneity.
	D	False	'Drop-outs' should be included in an 'intention to treat analysis'.
	E	True	See also *Companion to Psychiatric Studies*, page 186.

(Further details can be found in the *Companion to Psychiatric Studies*, pp. 152–154.)

5.4 With respect to research ethics:

A No study involving human subjects should start until approval of an independent ethics committee has been obtained.

B Informed consent must be obtained from a subject before undertaking any study-related procedures.

C It must be made clear to patients in writing that neither their current nor future treatment will be prejudiced if they withdraw from a study.

D Placebo-controlled studies are only justifiable if there is genuine uncertainty as to whether the treatment is better than placebo.

E Placebo-controlled studies are only justifiable if there is a reasonable possibility that the treatment will be better than placebo.

5.5 With respect to collecting data:

A Response rates to mailed questionnaires are usually less than 40%.

B It is important to collect as much data as possible from records.

C The General Health Questionnaire (GHQ) can be used to screen for psychotic illness.

D The Present State Examination is a structured mental state interview.

E The Schedule for Affective Disorders and Schizophrenia (SADS) is a structured interview.

5.6 When considering research data:

A In nominal categorical systems different individuals or objects are arranged in discrete mutually exclusive categories according to clearly defined characteristics.

B Different nominal categories are logically ordered.

C Different ordinal categories are logically ordered.

D Interval scales have a true zero point.

E Ratio scales have a true zero point.

(Answers overleaf)

5.4   A   **True**
       B   **True**
       C   **True**
       D   **True**
       E   **True**

(Further details can be found in the *Companion to Psychiatric Studies*, p. 154.)

5.5   A   **False**   The response rate tends to be 40–60%.
       B   **False**   Data tend to be incomplete and inaccurate.
       C   **False**   The GHQ is a screen for non-psychotic illness.
       D   **True**
       E   **False**   The SADS is semistructured.

(Further details can be found in the *Companion to Psychiatric Studies*, pp. 155–157.)

5.6   A   **True**
       B   **False**   Nominal data are not logically ordered.
       C   **True**
       D   **False**   Degrees Fahrenheit is an example.
       E   **True**   Weight in kilograms is an example.

(Further details can be found in the *Companion to Psychiatric Studies*, p. 158.)

5.7   With respect to psychiatric rating scales:

A   Rating scales are used to convert descriptive information into numerical data.

B   Scores on a rating scale should not be used to determine either inclusion into or exclusion from a study.

C   Rating scales work best in populations similar to those in which they were developed.

D   The Brief Psychiatric Rating Scale (BPRS) measures both positive and negative symptoms.

E   There are separate Hamilton Rating Scales for anxiety and depression.

5.8   Regarding the standard deviation (SD):

A   It is a measure of the spread of scores.

B   It is the sum of the squares of the differences between each score and the mean, divided by the total number of scores.

C   It should always be reported along with its respective mean.

D   It is always less than the mean.

E   In a normally distributed sample, 95% of scores lie within one standard deviation of the mean.

5.9   When using statistics to summarise data:

A   The standard error (SE) of the mean is a function of the standard deviation of the sample and of the sample size.

B   The standard error of the mean enables you to estimate the range within which the mean would probably fall if the study were repeated.

C   Confidence intervals can be readily calculated from the mean and standard error only if the variable is assumed to be normally distributed.

D   For a normally distributed variable, the probability of the population mean lying more than 2 standard errors away from the sample mean is less than 5%.

E   It is conventional to report 90% confidence intervals.

5.10   Inferential statistics:

A   Are concerned with hypothesis testing.

B   Can be used to prove that the null hypothesis is true.

C   Cannot demonstrate statistically significant effects.

D   Can be used to demonstrate that a result is important.

E   Help the researchers interpret their data.

(Answers overleaf)

5.7   **A**   **True**
     B   **False**   They can be so used.
     C   **True**
     D   **False**   The BPRS only measures positive symptoms.
     E   **True**   See also *Companion to Psychiatric Studies*, page 162.

(Further details can be found in the *Companion to Psychiatric Studies*, p. 159.)

5.8   **A**   **True**   Approximately, it is the mean deviation of all the scores from the mean.
     B   **False**   This is the variance, the square root of which is the standard deviation.
     C   **True**   It enables assessment of the position of a score relative to the mean.
     D   **False**   The SD is larger than the mean in extremely skewed data.
     E   **False**   95% of scores are within 1.96 standard deviations in the normal distribution.

(Further details can be found in the *Companion to Psychiatric Studies*, p. 166.)

5.9   **A**   **True**   Standard error is calculated as the SD divided by the square root of the sample size.
     B   **True**   About 68% of sample means will be ± 1 SE from the true mean.
     C   **True**
     D   **True**
     E   **False**   95% confidence intervals are generally reported.

(Further details can be found in the *Companion to Psychiatric Studies*, p. 167.)

5.10   **A**   **True**
     B   **False**   The null hypothesis can only be disproved (see also *Companion to Psychiatric Studies*, p. 190).
     C   **False**
     D   **False**   Statistical significance is not the same as clinical significance (see also *Companion to Psychiatric Studies*, p. 190).
     E   **True**

(Further details can be found in the *Companion to Psychiatric Studies*, pp. 168–169.)

5.11 **Parametric statistical tests rely upon the following assumptions:**
- A The population from which the sample is taken is normally distributed.
- B The groups being compared have similar means.
- C The groups being compared have similar standard deviations.
- D The scale of measurement is interval or ratio.
- E The scores within each sample are independent.

5.12 **Non-parametric statistical tests:**
- A Are less sensitive than their parametric counterparts.
- B Are unsuitable for handling ranked data.
- C Examine differences between medians rather than means.
- D Include the independent t test.
- E Include the chi-squared (χ^2) test.

5.13 **With respect to correlations:**
- A Correlation coefficients are always between 0 and 1.
- B A correlation coefficient above 0.7 suggests a strong causal link.
- C Transformation of data may allow non-linear correlations to be handled as linear.
- D Outliers may result in a correlation coefficient which is misleading.
- E If A is correlated with B and B is correlated with C then A is correlated with C.

5.14 **Survival analysis:**
- A Was originally developed as a statistical tool for predicting life expectancy.
- B Deals with the length of time elapsing before a particular event occurs.
- C Is incompatible with non-parametric data.
- D Predicts that a constant hazard rate will lead to a survival curve that is linear.
- E Results are often reported in terms of typical survival time.

(Answers overleaf)

5.11   **A** **True**
       B **False**   See C below.
       C **True**
       D **True**   Provided the means are approximately normally distributed.
       E **True**   This is the most important of all (see also *Companion to Psychiatric Studies*, p. 188).

(Further details can be found in the *Companion to Psychiatric Studies*, p. 170.)

5.12   **A** **True**
       B **False**   They are specifically for ranked data.
       C **True**
       D **False**   The *t* test is a parametric test.
       E **True**   The chi-squared test compares proportions on categorical measures.

(Further details can be found in the *Companion to Psychiatric Studies*, pp. 170–171 (including Table 5.7).)

5.13   **A** **False**   Correlations can be negative, i.e. the range is from −1 to 1.
       B **False**   Correlations measure association rather than causation.
       C **True**
       D **True**
       E **False**   It is not necessarily so.

(Further details can be found in the *Companion to Psychiatric Studies*, pp. 176–177.)

5.14   **A** **True**
       B **True**
       C **False**   Non-parametric data such as changes in occupation can be analysed.
       D **False**   A constant hazard rate produces an exponential survival curve.
       E **True**

(Further details can be found in the *Companion to Psychiatric Studies*, pp. 180–181.)

5.15 **When deciding how many subjects to recruit for a study:**

 A The number of subjects required is often far higher than clinicians might expect.

 B It is important to know the smallest effect that would be considered clinically valuable.

 C It is essential to perform a power calculation.

 D The number of groups in the study design is not important.

 E Too few subjects will result in an unacceptably high risk of a type 1 error occurring.

5.16 **When considering meta-analysis:**

 A The topic to be reviewed must be clearly defined from the outset.

 B It is best only to include studies that have been published in respected journals (e.g. those listed on MEDLINE or equivalent).

 C Publication bias can be evaluated using a funnel plot.

 D The double-blind randomised controlled trial is the gold standard experimental design.

 E All studies should be given equal weight.

(Answers overleaf)

5.15 A **True**
      B **True**
      C **True**
      D **False**
      E **False**   There is a high risk of type 2 error, i.e. a false negative.

(Further details can be found in the *Companion to Psychiatric Studies*, pp. 186–187.)

5.16 A **True**
      B **False**   This is prone to publication bias.
      C **True**
      D **True**
      E **False**   Larger studies should be given greater weight.

(Further details can be found in the *Companion to Psychiatric Studies*, pp. 191–192.)

6. Epidemiology

6.1 **Epidemiology:**
  A   Began as the study of epidemics.
  B   Was first put into practice by John Snow working on cholera in London.
  C   Was developed in the 1930s by Bradford Hill.
  D   Uses research principles that can be applied to almost any medical condition.
  E   In 1952, led to a randomised controlled trial (RCT) of streptomycin as a treatment for tuberculosis which was the first medical RCT ever conducted.

6.2 **Early triumphs of epidemiology include:**
  A   The discovery of penicillin.
  B   The pasteurisation of milk.
  C   A demonstration of the efficacy of streptomycin in tuberculosis.
  D   A demonstration of the association between smoking and lung cancer.
  E   The abolition of psychosurgery.

6.3 **When considering causes and mechanisms:**
  A   To establish the cause of a disease in humans, human populations must be studied.
  B   In vitro studies give clues about the mechanisms of diseases.
  C   Epidemiology is primarily concerned with the mechanism of disease.
  D   Epidemiological methods can be employed to test psychosocial but not biological aetiological hypotheses in psychiatry.
  E   The interplay between epidemiology and laboratory-based research is an important source of scientific advance in most medical fields.

(Answers overleaf)

6.1   A   True
     B   True
     C   True
     D   True   Epidemiology is defined as the quantitative population-based study of the aetiology, treatment and prevention of disease.
     E   True   Hill published the first randomised controlled trial in 1952.

(Further details can be found in the *Companion to Psychiatric Studies*, p. 197.)

6.2   A   False   This was a triumph for microbiology.
     B   False   See A above.
     C   True
     D   True
     E   False

(Further details can be found in the *Companion to Psychiatric Studies*, p. 197.)

6.3   A   True   Study of human populations is often a preliminary to laboratory research.
     B   True
     C   False   Its primary concern is the aetiology of disease.
     D   False   Both can be investigated.
     E   True

(Further details can be found in the *Companion to Psychiatric Studies*, pp. 197–198.)

6.4   **Within the field of epidemiology:**

A   The term 'outcome' is used as shorthand for the disease being observed.

B   The term 'exposure' is used as shorthand for the variable under investigation.

C   Between-observer variation is reduced by standardised, structured assessments.

D   Diseases are best viewed as present or absent rather than as a continuum.

E   A 'floating numerator' is of limited value.

6.5   **When measuring the frequency of a disease:**

A   Prevalence rates are a measure of new cases.

B   The incidence of a disease is determined using a cross-sectional survey.

C   Incidence is a proportion and can therefore be best expressed as a percentage.

D   With prevalence rates the denominator is person-time.

E   A chronic disease will have a high incidence but low prevalence.

6.6   **When using epidemiological measures of association:**

A   Relative risk gives an estimate of the 'aetiological force' of an exposure.

B   Standardised mortality ratios are commonly based on routinely collected data.

C   Relative risk for an exposure will be higher in a population which has a high base rate of a disease than in a population in which the disease is less common.

D   'Odds ratio' is another name for 'risk ratio'.

E   To make the results easier to interpret, odds ratios can be calculated both before and after adjustment for potential confounding variables.

(Answers overleaf)

6.4   A   **False**   'Disease' is the outcome of interest.
     B   **True**
     C   **True**
     D   **False**   Disease is best thought of as a continuum in epidemiology.
     E   **True**   One needs to know the denominator (see *Companion to Psychiatric Studies*, p.199).

(Further details can be found in the *Companion to Psychiatric Studies*, pp. 198–199.)

6.5   A   **False**
     B   **False**
     C   **False**
     D   **False**
     E   **False**

Note: All are true if 'prevalence' is substituted for 'incidence' and vice versa. (Further details can be found in the *Companion to Psychiatric Studies*, p. 199.)

6.6   A   **True**
     B   **True**
     C   **False**   The relative risk will be the same.
     D   **False**   Odds ratio is the ratio of odds; risk ratio is the ratio of prevalences.
     E   **True**

(Further details can be found in the *Companion to Psychiatric Studies*, p. 200.)

6.7   **With regard to the population attributable fraction:**

A   It is a measure of the importance of an aetiological agent in the population as a whole.

B   It is dependent on the relative risk and the frequency of exposure.

C   For it to be high, there must be both a large relative risk and a high rate of exposure.

D   Population attributable factors are used to plan disease-prevention strategies.

E   The population fraction for suicide attributable to unemployment is 10%; thus, eliminating unemployment should reduce the number of suicides by 10%.

6.8   **Study designs commonly used in epidemiological research include:**

A   Cross-sectional cohort surveys.

B   Case–control studies.

C   Ecological studies.

D   Randomised controlled trials.

E   Systematic reviews.

6.9   **Possible sources of bias in epidemiological studies include:**

A   Poor selection of controls.

B   The procedure of matching controls to individual cases.

C   Use of a measurement of exposure not independent of presence of disease.

D   Retrospective exposure assessment.

E   Effort after meaning.

6.10   **Ecological studies:**

A   Examine associations between disease and the characteristics of groups of people rather than characteristics of individuals.

B   Are inherently undermined by the 'ecological fallacy'.

C   Are relatively resistant to confounding factors.

D   Are able to examine the influence of sociological factors such as unemployment and deprivation upon incidence of illness.

E   Show that the more consultant psychiatrists there are in an area, the lower the suicide rate.

(Answers overleaf)

6.7   A   True
       B   True
       C   False   One or other is sufficient.
       D   True   They can inform how many cases are attributable to a
                     particular cause.
       E   True   This assumes that unemployment causes suicide.

(Further details can be found in the *Companion to Psychiatric Studies*, p. 201.)

6.8   A   False   Cohort studies are longitudinal.
       B   True
       C   True
       D   True
       E   True

(Further details can be found in the *Companion to Psychiatric Studies*, p. 201 (Table 6.1).)

6.9   A   True
       B   True
       C   True
       D   True
       E   True   It is the recall bias that can occur in ill people looking
                     for an explanation of illness.

(Further details can be found in the *Companion to Psychiatric Studies*, p. 203.)

6.10   A   True
       B   True   The exposure–disease association at population and
                     individual levels may differ.
       C   False   They are more susceptible to confounding than other
                     designs.
       D   True
       E   False   This is an example of an ecological fallacy; there are
                     more psychiatrists and more suicides in deprived
                     areas.

(Further details can be found in the *Companion to Psychiatric Studies*, pp. 204–205.)

6.11 **Regarding randomised controlled trials:**

A   They can be though of as matched cohort studies in which unknown confounders are randomly allocated.

B   They are observational studies.

C   A double-blind design eliminates the chance of measurement bias.

D   Subjects who drop out should be left out of the final analysis.

E   Provided the randomisation process is unbiased, it is not necessary to analyse the data for potentially confounding variables.

6.12 **Statistical power:**

A   Gives the probability that a type 1 error will not occur.

B   Depends upon the strength of the expected association in relation to the measurement error.

C   Depends upon the prevalence of the exposure.

D   Depends upon the significance level chosen.

E   Depends upon the sample size.

6.13 **Confounding variables in epidemiological research can be:**

A   Associated with both exposure and disease.

B   Either a risk factor or a protective factor.

C   Taken into account by introducing randomisation into a study design.

D   Taken into account by introducing matching into a study design.

E   On the causal pathway between exposure and disease.

6.14 **The following are ways of adjusting data sets for confounders during analysis:**

A   Randomisation.

B   Stratifying the sample by the confounding variable.

C   Logistic regression.

D   Least squares regression.

E   Residual confounding.

(Answers overleaf)

6.11 **A** **True**

B **False** They are experimental studies.
C **False** Blinding only reduces the chances of measurement bias.
D **False** Drop-outs should be considered in an intention to treat analysis.
F **False** Even unbiased randomisation can result in differences between the groups.

(Further details can be found in the *Companion to Psychiatric Studies*, p. 206.)

6.12 **A** **False** It gives the probability that a type 2 error will not occur.
B **True**
C **True**
D **True**
E **True**

As B, C, D, and E increase, the power of the study increases. (Further details can be found in the *Companion to Psychiatric Studies*, p. 208.)

6.13 **A** **True**
B **True**
C **True**
D **True**
E **False**

(Further details can be found in the *Companion to Psychiatric Studies*, p. 208.)

6.14 **A** **False** This limits confounding during study design.
B **True** The true relationship emerges in each stratum and the association is summarised by taking a weighted mean across the strata.
C **True** It is a multivariate technique for a binary outcome.
D **True** It is a multivariate technique for a continuous outcome.
E **False** Residual confounding is a descriptive term for uncontrolled confounding.

(Further details can be found in the *Companion to Psychiatric Studies*, pp. 208–210.)

7. Genetics

7.1 **Regarding chromosomes and cell division:**
  A   Chromosomes are visible under the microscope in the metaphase of cell division.
  B   The short arm of a chromosome is nominated the q arm.
  C   The centromere is of no significance to cell division.
  D   The telomeres prevent loss of DNA during replication.
  E   46 is the haploid count in human cells.

7.2 **The following are true of cell division:**
  A   In mitosis, chromosomes are duplicated during the prophase of the cell cycle.
  B   Recombination is the initial phase of establishing an individual's molecular identity.
  C   The recombination rate is the physical basis of linkage analysis.
  D   The second meiotic cell division involves duplication of chromosomal material.
  E   In the formation of ova all of the four gametes survive to produce an ovum.

(Answers overleaf)

7.1   **A True**   The chromosomes are most compact during metaphase and are visible under the microscope.

B False   Each chromosome is divided into a long (q) and short (p) arm by the centromere.

C False   The centromere attaches itself to the spindle apparatus and plays a major role in chromosome assortment during cell division.

D True   The chromosome ends, the telomeres, are functionally specialised, stabilising the chromosome and preventing loss of DNA during replication.

E False   Most human cells have 44 autosomes and two sex chromosomes (the diploid count of 46); while sperm and ova have the haploid count of 23 chromosomes.

(Further details can be found in the *Companion to Psychiatric Studies*, p. 219.)

7.2   **A True**   Somatic cells divide by mitosis in which each chromosome is duplicated during the prophase of the cell cycle; gamete formation is by meiosis.

B True   Recombination is the first of three essential processes (recombination, random assortment of chromosomes at fertilisation and DNA mutations) that establish the molecular individuality of an individual.

C. True   Recombination rate can be used as an estimate of the distances between two points on a chromosome as the greater the physical distance between two markers the more likely they are to be separated during meiosis; it is the physical basis of linkage analysis.

D False   Meiosis proceeds to a second meiotic cell division without duplication of chromosomal material, producing four gametes with a haploid count of chromosomes.

E False   In the formation of ova only one of the four gametes survives as an ovum, the others form polar bodies.

(Further details can be found in the *Companion to Psychiatric Studies*, p. 219.)

7.3   **Regarding the DNA in chromosomes:**

A   The complementary pairing of bases in DNA includes adenine to cytosine.

B   30% of human genes on each chromosome may be related to the development and function of the CNS.

C   Genes are evenly shared between chromosomes.

D   Tandem repeats of nucleotides constitute only the minority of human DNA sequences.

E   The total number of repeats in a block is inherited stably.

7.4   **Concerning deletion:**

A   Examples of gene dosage anomalies include partial monosomies and trisomies.

B   Velocardiofacial syndrome is an example of a microdeletion.

C   Unstable triplet repeats can result in neuropsychiatric conditions.

D   Huntington's disease is caused by triplet repeats outwith the coding region.

E   Myotonic dystrophy is caused by triplet repeats within the coding region.

7.5   **Regarding recessive patterns of inheritance:**

A   Consanguinity in a family can result in rare recessive disorders being over-represented.

B   Cystic fibrosis affects 1 in 2500 live births.

C   If both parents are heterozygous for a gene then, on average, one in four children will be affected.

D   In recessive conditions there must be evidence of cases in previous generations.

E   Recessive conditions affect approximately 10 per 1000 live births.

(Answers overleaf)

7.3   **A** **False**   Complementary base pairing is adenine to thymine and cytosine to guanine.

        B **True**   Each chromosome has on average 130 million base pairs and will contain around 4000 genes, 30% of which may be related to the development and function of the CNS.

        C **False**   Genes are not evenly shared between chromosomes.

        D **False**   Most DNA does not have a known coding function but includes stretches of repeat sequence nucleotides, known as tandem repeats.

        E **True**   The total number of repeats and the overall size of the block is highly variable in the population but is stably inherited.

(Further details can be found in the *Companion to Psychiatric Studies*, p. 220.)

7.4   **A** **True**

        B **True**   DiGeorge syndrome is another example.

        C **True**   Unstable triplet repeats are duplication mutations that cause several neuropsychiatric conditions.

        D **False**   Repeats *within* the coding regions cause Huntington's disease and the spinocerebellar ataxias.

        E **False**   Triplet repeats *outwith* the coding frame cause myotonic dystrophy and Friedreich's ataxia.

(Further details can be found in the *Companion to Psychiatric Studies*, p. 221.)

7.5   **A** **True**   There is often an increased rate of consanguinity in families expressing a rare recessive disorder.

        B **True**

        C **True**   If both parents have one copy of the mutant gene then, on average, one in four of their children will be affected.

        D **False**   There may be no evidence of any other cases in previous generations and the disease may apparently only appear in children.

        E **False**   Overall, recessive conditions are rare, affecting 2–3 per 1000 live births.

(Further details can be found in the *Companion to Psychiatric Studies*, pp. 221–222 and Fig. 7.1, p. 223.)

7.6   **Regarding dominant and sex-linked patterns of inheritance:**

   A   Dominant disorders tend to show vertical inheritance.

   B   Half of the sibship tends to be affected in dominant conditions.

   C   Penetrance of a condition is the proportion of homozygotes expressing the condition.

   D   In X-linked conditions there is male-to-male vertical inheritance.

   E   Affected males are more common in X-linked pedigrees.

7.7   **Concerning patterns of inheritance generally:**

   A   Epistasis refers to gene–gene interaction influencing the expression of phenotype.

   B   A proportion of presenile familial dementia of Alzheimer's type is caused by one gene mutation.

   C   ApoE gene alleles show no epistatic effect and lead directly to late-onset dementia.

   D   There can be only one pathogenic mutation within one single gene.

   E   Psychiatric disorders cannot be investigated using techniques similar to those uncovering the genetic basis of physical conditions such as breast cancer.

(Answers overleaf)

7.6 A True Dominant conditions, on average, affect subjects in all generations – 'vertical inheritance'.

B True

C False The penetrance of a condition is the proportion of people with a mutated gene on one chromosome, i.e. heterozygotes, showing any feature of the disease.

D False Males can only pass on their Y chromosome to their sons so there is no male-to-male vertical inheritance in X-linked conditions but affected males are more common in X-linked pedigrees.

E True

(Further details can be found in the *Companion to Psychiatric Studies*, p. 222 and Fig. 7.1, p. 223.)

7.7 A True Epistasis refers to one gene interacting with another gene on the same or a different chromosome to influence the genotype.

B False A proportion of presenile familial dementia of Alzheimer's type can be caused independently by mutations in three different genes.

C False Specific alleles of ApoE have the epistatic effect of increasing risk of or protecting against the development of dementia.

D False In addition to one disease arising from mutations in many different genes, there may be a host of different pathogenic mutations within one single gene.

E False There are as yet no reasons why psychiatric syndromes should be less amenable to genetic investigation than their physical counterparts.

(Further details can be found in the *Companion to Psychiatric Studies*, p. 222.)

7.8   **With regard to the phenomena of anticipation and imprinting:**

A   Anticipation has been described in bipolar disorder.

B   Triplet repeat expansion has been found in bipolar disorder and explains the existence of anticipation in this condition.

C   Parent of origin effects are due to imprinting of genes in the germline.

D   Imprinting affects both genotype and phenotype.

E   Uniparental disomy is a form of imprinting.

7.9   **Regarding family studies:**

A   First-degree relatives share, on average, 25% of their genes.

B   Rates of affective disorder and schizophrenia are higher in relatives of affected probands than in normal controls.

C   Segregation analysis is the method whereby comparison is made between observed and expected proportions of relatives affected.

D   Dominant and recessive patterns have been described for psychiatric illnesses.

E   No X-linked pedigree for major mental illness has, as yet, been described.

(Answers overleaf)

7.8   **A**   **True**   Anticipation is the phenomenon whereby a disease has an earlier age of onset and increased severity in succeeding generations. This has been described in bipolar disorder.

      B   **False**   Triplet repeat expansion, the basis of anticipation in fragile X syndrome, has not been found convincingly in the major psychoses.

      C   **True**   Parent of origin effects occur where different phenotypes are associated with paternal and maternal inheritance of a disorder. The mechanism of the effect is thought to lie in the differential contribution of genes from each parent through so-called imprinting of genes in the germline.

      D   **False**   Imprinting affects phenotype but not genotype.

      E   **True**   Imprinting is seen in fragile X, Prader–Willi and Angelman syndromes and in uniparental disomy, where both chromosomes are inherited from one parent.

(Further details can be found in the *Companion to Psychiatric Studies*, pp. 222–224.)

7.9   **A**   **False**   First-degree relatives share an average of 50% of their genes.

      B   **True**   Rates of affective disorders, schizophrenia, anxiety disorders, personality disorders and a range of behaviours are higher in relatives of affected probands.

      C   **True**

      D   **True**   Psychiatric illnesses may well be genetically heterogeneous and families showing apparent dominant, recessive and X-linked patterns have been described.

      E   **False**   See D above.

(Further details can be found in the *Companion to Psychiatric Studies*, p. 225.)

7.10 **With regard to adoption studies:**

A   Parent as proband adoption studies have failed to show any evidence of a genetic basis for schizophrenia.

B   The Danish adoption study of schizophrenia used the adoptee as proband technique.

C   In utero environmental influences can confound adoption studies.

D   Cross-fostering design compares rates of illness in one group of children fostered out to different parents.

E   Adoption studies of children adopted shortly after birth are free from confounds.

7.11 **Concerning twin studies:**

A   Dizygotic twins are genetically more similar than non-twin siblings.

B   Concordance rate measures the phenotypic similarity between twins.

C   Pair-wise concordance is the number of affected co-twins of an affected proband divided by the total number of co-twins in the study.

D   Proband-wise concordance is more commonly quoted in the literature than pair-wise concordance.

E   Proband-wise and pair-wise are two methods of gaining the same result.

(Answers overleaf)

7.10 **A** **False** The Oregon Schizophrenia Study (Heston 1966) used a parent as proband technique and found that there was a significant increase in schizophrenia in the adoptees whose mothers were schizophrenic compared to controls.

B **True**

C **True** A criticism of adoption studies is that they cannot exclude the possibility of strong shared environmental influences in utero.

D **False** Cross-fostering design compares rate of illness in two groups of adoptees: one with ill parents and adopted by well parents; the other with well biological parents but brought up in a family where one parent has become ill.

E **False** Children adopted shortly after birth will still have experienced the prenatal and perinatal environment of their biological mother and after adoption may suffer greater stress by virtue of being an adoptee.

(Further details can be found in the *Companion to Psychiatric Studies*, p. 225.)

7.11 **A** **False** Dizygotic twins are no more alike genetically than normal siblings.

B **True** Concordance rates measure the similarity of phenotype between twins.

C **False** Pair-wise concordance is the number of pairs of twins where both are affected divided by the total number of pairs studied.

D **True** The proband-wise concordance, i.e. the number of affected co-twins of an affected proband divided by the total number co-twins in the study, is more commonly quoted in the literature.

E **False** Proband-wise concordance will be different from pair-wise because some twins will be counted twice if they have been independently ascertained.

(Further details can be found in the *Companion to Psychiatric Studies*, pp. 225–226.)

7.12   **The following are true of twin studies:**
   A   Environmental influences, by definition, do not include genetic effects.
   B   There is no apparent genetic contribution to panic disorder.
   C   They have been informative in measuring the size of the genetic contribution to sexual orientation.
   D   There is no difference in the intraclass correlation between monozygotic and dizygotic in a highly genetic disease.
   E   The Minnesota Twin Study provides an estimate of variance due to genetic factors using within-pair correlations.

7.13   **With respect to linkage analysis:**
   A   Small family collections are of no use in linkage studies.
   B   Sibling pair analysis is the only effective technique in linkage analysis.
   C   Linkage analysis exploits the characteristic of all chromosomes to recombine during meiosis.
   D   Recombination on average occurs at one stretch of DNA every two meioses.
   E   Rates of recombination are measured in centimorgans.

(Answers overleaf)

7.12   **A**   **False**   Environmental influences include non-transmitted genetic effects, e.g. somatic mutations, repeat sequence expansion and variation in methylation, which could affect the expression of inherited genetic factors.

   B   **False**   Family and twin studies have established evidence for a substantial genetic contribution to schizophrenia and bipolar disorder, and a weaker but important contribution to panic, alcoholism and anorexia.

   C   **True**   Twin studies have been informative in measuring the genetic contribution to nearly all aspects of behaviour, including personality, cognitive abilities and sexual orientation.

   D   **False**   For a variable under strong genetic influence, the intraclass correlation will be higher between monozygotic than dizygotic twins.

   E   **True**   The Minnesota Twin Study provides an estimate of variance due to genetic factors using within-pair correlations – an unusual chance to study the effects of nature and nurture.

(Further details can be found in the *Companion to Psychiatric Studies*, p. 226.)

7.13   **A**   **False**   Very large pedigrees or collections of smaller families where the effect of linkage is additive are studied in linkage analysis.

   B   **False**   Studying pairs of affected siblings is only one of a number of approaches.

   C   **True**

   D   **False**   Recombination occurs when homologous chromosomes pair up during meiosis and exchange stretches of DNA, i.e. at about two stretches of DNA on each chromosome every meiosis.

   E   **True**   The statistical unit to describe rates of recombination is the centimorgan.

(Further details can be found in the *Companion to Psychiatric Studies*, p. 227.)

7.14   **Concerning recombination:**

    A   Independent assortment is ensured by recombination.

    B   The further apart a polymorphic marker is for a disease locus, the more often the two will remain together from generation to generation.

    C   In a mating, if a marker and a disease become separated then recombination has occurred.

    D   The recombination fraction equals the number of recombinants divided by the total number of offspring.

    E   The recombination fraction is proportional to the physical distance, whether long or short, between two loci.

7.15   **Regarding linkage analysis:**

    A   Genes on two different chromosomes have a one in four chance of remaining together during meiosis and thus being transmitted to the offspring.

    B   LOD score is the statistical method used for calculating linkage.

    C   LOD is the logarithm of the odds that the recombination fraction has a value, divided by the odds that the value is 0.5.

    D   LOD score of 3 is conventionally accepted as evidence of linkage.

    E   LOD score of 0 is accepted as excluding linkage.

(Answers overleaf)

7.14 **A** **True** Recombination ensures a mixing of genetic material so that two traits that are physically far apart on a chromosome or on different chromosomes will assort independently.

B **False** In general, the closer a polymorphic marker is to a disease locus the more often the two will remain together from one generation to the next.

C **True**
D **True**
E **False** The recombination fraction is proportional to the physical distance between two loci over short distances only.

(Further details can be found in the *Companion to Psychiatric Studies*, pp. 227–228.)

7.15 **A** **False** Genes on different chromosomes or far apart on the same chromosome cosegregate randomly and have a 50:50 chance of remaining together during meiosis and being transmitted to offspring.

B **True** The conventional statistical method of testing for linkage is to calculate the LOD score from the recombination fraction, i.e. the common logarithm of the odds that the recombination fraction has a value, divided by the odds that the value is 0.5.

C **True** See B above.
D **True** It is conventionally accepted that a LOD score of 3 (odds in favour 1000:1) is proof of linkage and LOD of –2 (odds against of 100:1) is proof of exclusion.

E **False** See D above.

(Further details can be found in the *Companion to Psychiatric Studies*, pp. 227–228.)

8. Psychiatric interviewing

8.1 **The functions described in the Three Function Model of interviewing are:**
  A   Gathering data to understand the patient.
  B   Development of rapport.
  C   Clarification of the transference.
  D   Making a diagnosis.
  E   Patient education and behavioural management.

8.2 **Influential models in medical interviewing include:**
  A   The biopsychosocial approach.
  B   The Three Function Model.
  C   The Patient-Centred Clinical Method.
  D   Potter's intensive programme.
  E   Multivariate regression.

8.3 **The patient-centred approach:**
  A   Was the subject matter of a book titled *Meetings Between Patients* by Tuckett.
  B   Involves sitting the person in the middle of the family.
  C   Emphasises the importance of the patient's own view of the problem.
  D   Means all patients should be seen in primary care.
  E   Is a form of alternative medicine.

8.4 **The following are open-ended questions:**
  A   How are you?
  B   What is wrong?
  C   Do you have pain?
  D   What is the date?
  E   Are you constipated?

8.5 **When assessing a potentially violent patient, it is advisable to:**
  A   Meet aggression with aggression.
  B   Remain standing.
  C   Ensure that a third person is present in the room at all times.
  D   Freely express your own feeling of anger.
  E   Limit the interview to 10 minutes.

(Answers overleaf)

8.1 A True
       B True
       C False
       D False
       E True

(Further details can be found in the *Companion to Psychiatric Studies*, p. 234.)

8.2 A True
       B True
       C True
       D False
       E False

(Further details can be found in the *Companion to Psychiatric Studies*, p. 234.)

8.3 A False The title of the book is *Meetings Between Experts*.
       B False
       C True
       D False
       E False

(Further details can be found in the *Companion to Psychiatric Studies*, p. 234.)

8.4 A False
       B True
       C False
       D False
       E False

(Further details can be found in the *Companion to Psychiatric Studies*, p. 236.)

8.5 A False Remain calm without expressing feelings.
       B False It is essential that both parties sit down.
       C False A third person should be outside the room within calling distance.
       D False Do not express your own feelings.
       E False Allow considerable time.

(Further details can be found in the *Companion to Psychiatric Studies*, p. 238.)

8.6   **Key elements of motivational interviewing include:**

    A   Criticising the problem behaviour repeatedly.

    B   Clarifying the patient's view of the problem.

    C   Listing to the pros and cons of the behaviour.

    D   Providing information.

    E   Relieving the patient of responsibility for his or her actions.

(Answers overleaf)

8.6   A   **False**   Remain neutral.
      B   **True**
      C   **True**
      D   **True**   For example, information about risks of the behaviour can be provided.
      E   **False**

(Further details can be found in the *Companion to Psychiatric Studies*, p. 244.)

9. Mental state examination

9.1 The following movement disorders occur in patients with schizophrenia:
A Waxy flexibility.
B Negativism.
C Mannerisms.
D Schnauzkrampf.
E Dysmegalopsia.

9.2 Characteristic features of flight of ideas include:
A Pressured speech.
B Clang association.
C Perseveration.
D Neologisms.
E Lack of association between elements of speech.

9.3 The following occur in schizophrenic thought disorder:
A Metonyms.
B Loosening of associations.
C Derailment.
D Neologisms.
E Thought blocking.

9.4 Anxiety:
A Is characteristically associated with a sense of threat.
B Is always pathological.
C Always leads to avoidance of the object of anxiety.
D Commonly leads to psychomotor retardation.
E Is often associated with autonomic arousal.

(Answers overleaf)

9.1   A   True   Patients' limbs remain in the position in which they were placed.
       B   True   Patients do the opposite of what they are told.
       C   True   These are repetitive purposeful movements.
       D   True   The patient's rounded lips are thrust forward.
       E   False   It is a distortion of vision associated with neurological disease.

(Further details can be found in the *Companion to Psychiatric Studies*, p. 250.)

9.2   A   True
       B   True   Clang association refers to the linkage of two words with a similar sound.
       C   False   Perseveration is repeated movement characteristic of frontal lobe lesions.
       D   False   They may be a feature of schizophrenic thought disorder.
       E   False   It is typical of schizophrenic thought disorder.

(Further details can be found in the *Companion to Psychiatric Studies*, p. 251.)

9.3   A   True   Metonyms are imprecise approximations for a more exact word.
       B   True
       C   True   Derailment is another name for loosening of associations.
       D   True   Neologisms are new idiosyncratic words.
       E   True   Thought blocking is sudden cessation in speech when the patient's mind 'becomes empty'.

(Further details can be found in the *Companion to Psychiatric Studies*, p. 251.)

9.4   A   True
       B   False
       C   False
       D   False
       E   True

(Further details can be found in the *Companion to Psychiatric Studies*, p. 252.)

9.5   **Elevated mood:**
A   Is usually acknowledged as pathological by the individual.
B   Is usually associated with a sense of well-being.
C   Always leads to increased activity and efficiency.
D   Only occurs in mania.
E   May present as irritability.

9.6   **The following are characteristic of depressive illness:**
A   Flattening of affect.
B   Affective blunting.
C   Anhedonia.
D   Negativism.
E   Incongruous affect.

9.7   **Primary delusions:**
A   May be autochthonous.
B   May take the form of a delusional perception.
C   Are understandable in terms of preceding morbid experiences.
D   Are often preceded by delusional mood.
E   Are always false.

9.8   **Schneider's 'first-rank' symptoms of schizophrenia:**
A   Are pathognomonic of schizophrenia.
B   Must be present for a diagnosis of schizophrenia.
C   Can be diagnosed reliably cross-culturally.
D   Are of prognostic value.
E   May occur in affective disorders.

(Answers overleaf)

9.5 A **False** It is often not recognised as such.
  B **True**
  C **True** Distractibility leads to inefficiency.
  D **False** It also occurs in organic states.
  E **True**

(Further details can be found in the *Companion to Psychiatric Studies*, p. 252.)

9.6 A **False** The term relates to schizophrenia.
  B **False** The term relates to schizophrenia.
  C **True** Anhedonia is loss of interest and pleasure.
  D **False** It occurs in schizophrenia.
  E **False** There are various causes.

(Further details can be found in the *Companion to Psychiatric Studies*, p. 252.)

9.7 A **True** They arise suddenly and fully formed.
  B **True** A new meaning and significance is attached to a specific perception.
  C **False** By definition, they arise de novo.
  D **True** The person feels that the world has changed in a perplexing way.
  E **False** The process of logic is in error – the belief is not necessarily false.

(Further details can be found in the *Companion to Psychiatric Studies*, p. 254.)

9.8 A **False** They are not pathognomonic – they can occur in affective and organic psychosis.
  B **False** They are not essential.
  C **True**
  D **False** They have no prognostic value.
  E **True** They can be symptoms of affective disorders, especially mania.

(Further details can be found in the *Companion to Psychiatric Studies*, p. 255.)

9.9   Schneider's 'first-rank' symptoms include:

A   Somatic passivity.
B   Thought broadcasting.
C   Thought echo.
D   Third person auditory hallucinations.
E   Primary delusions.

9.10   The following abnormalities of perception require a real perceptual object:

A   Dysmegalopsia.
B   Pareidolia.
C   Formication.
D   Reflex hallucination.
E   Synaesthesia.

9.11   With respect to consciousness:

A   A vigilant patient is always lucid.
B   Vigilance is largely controlled by the ascending reticular activating system.
C   Clouding of consciousness is characteristic of dementia.
D   Disorientation only occurs when consciousness is clouded.
E   Disorientation in time occurs only in severe cognitive impairment.

9.12   With respect to short-term memory:

A   Items can be retained for only 5 seconds.
B   Its capacity is limited to an average of seven items.
C   Its span can be extended by conscious rehearsal.
D   Impairment can lead to confabulation.
E   It is assessed by questions concerning recent news events.

(Answers overleaf)

9.9
  A True
  B True
  C True
  D True
  E True

(Further details can be found in the *Companion to Psychiatric Studies*, pp. 255–258.)

9.10
  A True   Dysmegalopsia is distortion in shape of a perception.
  B True   There are elaborate illusions from a simple stimulus.
  C False This is a somatic hallucination attributed to infestation.
  D False Real sensation in one modality leads to sensation in another.
  E False Synaesthesia is a type of hallucination.

(Further details can be found in the *Companion to Psychiatric Studies*, pp. 257–258.)

9.11
  A False But a lucid patient is always vigilant.
  B True
  C False It is characteristic of delirium.
  D False Disorientation also occurs in mental handicap and dementia.
  E False It is more easily disturbed than disorientation in place and person.

(Further details can be found in the *Companion to Psychiatric Studies*, pp. 258–259.)

9.12
  A False Items can be retained for only 30 seconds, unless rehearsed.
  B True
  C True
  D False This is true of impairment of long-term memory.
  E False It is assessed by the digit span test.

(Further details can be found in the *Companion to Psychiatric Studies*, pp. 259–260.)

9.13 **In psychogenic stupor, the patient:**

A   Is mute.
B   May be manic.
C   Is amnesic for events during stupor.
D   Exhibits clouding of consciousness.
E   Exhibits automatic obedience.

9.14 **Inability to name an object correctly may be due to:**

A   Nominal dysphasia.
B   Prosopagnosia.
C   Idiomotor apraxia.
D   Astereognosia.
E   Visual agnosia.

(Answers overleaf)

9.13 A **True**
      B **True**   Stupor is rarely associated with manic illness.
      C **False**   The patient is amnesic only in stupor of neurological origin.
      D **False**
      E **False**

(Further details can be found in the *Companion to Psychiatric Studies*, pp. 261–262.)

9.14 A **True**   The patient is unable to name an object but can talk about it.
      B **False**   Prosopagnosia is the inability to recognise faces.
      C **False**   Idiomotor apraxia is the inability to complete complex tasks on instruction.
      D **True**   It is the inability to identify a three-dimensional object by touch.
      E **True**   It is the inability to comprehend the significance of a visual stimulus.

(Further details can be found in the *Companion to Psychiatric Studies*, pp. 262–263.)

10. Diagnosis

10.1 **DSM-IV:**
A Was published in 1987.
B Has six axes.
C Records general medical as well as psychiatric diagnoses.
D Avoids operational definitions.
E Is identical to ICD-10.

10.2 **ICD-10:**
A Came into use in 1983.
B Uses an alphanumeric format.
C Categorises depressive disorders in both neurotic and psychotic sections.
D Categorises alcohol disorders in a separate section from other substances of misuse.
E Follows the operational definitions introduced in ICD-9.

10.3 **The following statements about the DSM classification are true:**
A The first edition was published in 1929.
B The third edition was only a minor modification of the second edition
C Axis V of DSM-III records lowest level of functioning in the past year.
D DSM-III discarded the term neurosis.
E Axis IV of DSM-III records social support.

10.4 **Reliability of psychiatric diagnosis:**
A Was established as high in Beck and Kreitman's 1960s studies.
B Is overestimated by the observer method of assessment.
C Is reduced by detailed operational definitions.
D Is best with unstructured interviews.
E Is lower for organic disorders than for neuroses.

(Answers overleaf)

10.1 A **False** That was DSM-IIIR; DSM-IV was published in 1994.
     B **False** It has five axes.
     C **True** It records general medical conditions on Axis III.
     D **False** It is based on operational definitions.
     E **False** Unfortunately there are significant differences.

(Further details can be found in the *Companion to Psychiatric Studies*, pp. 270–271.)

10.2 A **False** It came into use in 1993.
     B **True** It uses a mixture of letters and numbers in coding.
     C **False** They are grouped together as affective disorders (F3).
     D **False** They are together in disorders due to psychoactive substances (F1).
     E **False** ICD-9 was not an operational classification.

(Further details can be found in the *Companion to Psychiatric Studies*, pp. 273–274.)

10.3 A **False** It was published in 1952.
     B **False** It was radically different – it included operational definitions.
     C **False** It records highest level of functioning.
     D **True**
     E **False** It records severity of psychosocial stressors.

(Further details can be found in the *Companion to Psychiatric Studies*, pp. 274–275.)

10.4 A **False** It was established as low.
     B **True** A second rater rates the same interview; cf. interviewing again (reinterview method).
     C **False** Reliability is improved.
     D **False** Reliability is better with standardised interviews.
     E **False** Reliability is better for organic disorders.

(Further details can be found in the *Companion to Psychiatric Studies*, pp. 275–276.)

10.5   The validity of psychiatric diagnosis:

A   Is independent of reliability.

B   Is supported by the lack of specificity of psychiatric treatments.

C   Can be supported by cluster analysis.

D   Is refuted by family studies of schizophrenia.

E   Is measured by Cronbach's alpha.

10.6   Categorical methods of classification:

A   Do not imply unproven quantitative differences between patients.

B   Are more flexible than dimensions.

C   Were proposed by Eysenck.

D   Readily encompass the 'atypical'.

E   Are useful for guiding treatment.

(Answers overleaf)

10.5 A **False** Reliability limits validity.
     B **False** Its validity is supported by specificity of treatments, e.g. lithium.
     C **True** Cluster analysis is a statistical technique demonstrating clustering of symptoms.
     D. **False** The tendency to breed true is supportive.
     E **False** This is a statistical measure of scale reliability.

(Further details can be found in the *Companion to Psychiatric Studies*, pp. 276–277.)

10.6 A **False** They do imply unproven quantitative differences between patients.
     B **False** Dimensions can be recategorised at various levels.
     C **False** He proposed dimensional classification of personality.
     D **False** Atypical cases are a problem for categorical classifications.
     E **True**

(Further details can be found in the *Companion to Psychiatric Studies*, pp. 277–279.)

11. Organic disorders

11.1   **The following features are suggestive of a temporal lobe lesion:**
A   Contralateral upper quadrantic visual field lesions.
B   Contralateral hemiparesis.
C   Gerstmann's syndrome.
D   Dyspraxia.
E   Grasp reflex.

11.2   **The following features are especially suggestive of delirium:**
A   Overactivity.
B   Disorientation.
C   Fluctuating symptom level.
D   Delusional ideation.
E   Insidious onset of symptoms.

11.3   **The following are common causes of dementia in the UK.**
A   Wilson's disease.
B   Alzheimer's disease.
C   Alcohol abuse.
D   Pick's disease.
E   Huntington's disease.

11.4   **The following are true of Alzheimer's disease:**
A   The prevalence is about 10% in patients in their 80s.
B   It is the commonest single cause of dementia in the UK.
C   It is clinically easily distinguishable from Lewy body dementia.
D   It occurs with reduced frequency in patients with Down's syndrome.
E   Cigarette smoking is associated with increased risk of developing the disease.

11.5   **The following features occurring in presenile dementia raise the possibility of new variant CJD:**
A   Initial presentation with apparently non-organic psychiatric problems.
B   Cerebellar ataxia.
C   Urinary incontinence.
D   Onset before age 40.
E   Ophthalmoplegia.

(Answers overleaf)

11.1 A **True**
    B **True**
    C **False** Gerstmann's syndrome is a form of body image
            disturbance characteristic of parietal lesions.
    D **False** The association is with parietal lesions.
    E **False** The association is with frontal lesions.

(Further details can be found in the *Companion to Psychiatric Studies*, pp. 283–284.)

11.2 A **False** Overactivity is found in many psychiatric disorders.
    B **True**
    C **True**
    D **False** Delusional ideation is found in any type of psychosis.
    E **False** Symptoms are usually of sudden onset.

(Further details can be found in the *Companion to Psychiatric Studies*, pp. 286–287.)

11.3 A **False**
    B **True**
    C **True**
    D **False**
    E **False**

(Further details can be found in the *Companion to Psychiatric Studies*, p. 290.)

11.4 A **True**
    B **True**
    C **False** They may only be clearly differentiated at
            postmortem.
    D **False** It occurs with increased frequency.
    E **False** There is some evidence for reduced risk.

(Further details can be found in the *Companion to Psychiatric Studies*, p. 291.)

11.5 A **True**
    B **True**
    C **False**
    D **True**
    E **False**

(Further details can be found in the *Companion to Psychiatric Studies*, pp. 306–307.)

11.6 **Wernicke–Korsakoff syndrome is characterised by:**
A Medial frontal lobe damage.
B Nystagmus.
C Impaired recall of information.
D Ataxia.
E Paralysis of conjugate gaze.

11.7 **Postconcussional syndrome:**
A Is characterised by poor concentration.
B Usually persists at least 6 months.
C Following industrial accidents is likely to be worsened by litigation.
D Is associated with premorbid social problems.
E Is more likely to persist in women.

11.8 **The following are true of epilepsy:**
A Approximately 50% of patients with temporal lobe epilepsy have mesial temporal lobe sclerosis.
B 'Spike and wave' discharge on EEG is characteristic of simple absence seizures.
C Speech during a seizure suggests a temporal lobe focus.
D Conscious level is almost always altered during epileptic automatism.
E Simple partial seizures are usually of unknown causation.

11.9 **The following are more suggestive of epileptic seizures than non-epileptic attacks:**
A Stereotyped movements.
B Up-going plantar reflexes.
C Faecal incontinence.
D Opisthotonos.
E Asymmetric limb movements.

11.10 **Regarding depression following cerebrovascular accident (CVA):**
A There is an association with the size of the lesion.
B Depression is more common with temporal lobe lesions.
C Depression occurs in at least one-third of patients 6 months after CVA.
D Level of cognitive impairment correlates with depression.
E Life events have been shown to be predictive of depression following CVA.

(Answers overleaf)

11.6 A **False** Damage is to the temporal lobe.
B **True** It occurs in the acute phase.
C **True** It is characteristic of the chronic phase.
D **True** It occurs in the acute phase.
E **True** It occurs in the acute phase.

(Further details can be found in the *Companion to Psychiatric Studies*, pp. 307–308.)

11.7 A **True**
B **False** Usually, it persists only weeks to months.
C **False**
D **True**
E **True**

(Further details can be found in the *Companion to Psychiatric Studies*, p. 313.)

11.8 A **True**
B **True**
C **False** Frontal seizure is associated with phonation.
D **True**
E **False** They usually arise from a structural lesion.

(Further details can be found in the *Companion to Psychiatric Studies*, pp. 315–316.)

11.9 A **False**
B **True**
C **False**
D **False**
E **False**

(Further details can be found in the *Companion to Psychiatric Studies*, p. 318.)

11.10 A **True** The association is weak.
B **False**
C **False** It occurs in 13–34% of patients.
D **True**
E **False**

(Further details can be found in the *Companion to Psychiatric Studies*, p. 319.)

11.11   **The following are common psychiatric presentations of multiple sclerosis:**
A   Dysmnesic syndrome.
B   Low mood.
C   Persecutory delusions.
D   Confusion.
E   Personality change.

11.12   **Characteristic features of normal pressure hydrocephalus include:**
A   Onset in the second decade of life.
B   Disturbance of gait.
C   Cognitive impairment.
D   Pathognomonic EEG changes.
E   Urinary incontinence.

11.13   **The following are correctly paired:**
A   Persistent glabellar tap – frontal lobe lesion.
B   Sensory inattention – parietal lobe lesion.
C   Kayser–Fleischer rings – Wilson's disease.
D   Hypersomnolence – diencephalic lesion.
E   Hyperorality – Klüver–Bucy syndrome

11.14   **Huntington's disease has the following characteristics:**
A   It is X-linked.
B   Pathological findings typically include marked temporal lobe atrophy.
C   25% of patients show behavioural disturbance prior to manifesting neurological signs or symptoms.
D   The mean age of onset is 40.
E   Prenatal testing is available.

(Answers overleaf)

11.11   A   False
             B   True
             C   False
             D   False
             E   True

(Further details can be found in the *Companion to Psychiatric Studies*, p. 320.)

11.12   A   False   Onset is usually in the 60s and 70s.
             B   True
             C   True
             D   False
             E   True   Early incontinence is a useful pointer to this diagnosis.

(Further details can be found in the *Companion to Psychiatric Studies*, p. 305.)

11.13   A   False
             B   True
             C   True
             D   True
             E   True

(Further details can be found in the *Companion to Psychiatric Studies*, pp. 283–300.)

11.14   A   False   The pattern of inheritance is autosomal dominant.
             B   False   Cortical atrophy is prominent in the frontal lobes.
             C   False   40% have prodromal behaviour disorders, e.g. aggression.
             D   True
             E   True

(Further details can be found in the *Companion to Psychiatric Studies*, pp. 303–304.)

12. Substance misuse

12.1   Kreitman's alcohol misuse prevention paradox:
A   Suggests that alcohol prevention measures should be focused on heavy drinkers.
B   Indicates that prevention strategies for heavy drinkers will have less beneficial impact on society than prevention strategies for less heavy drinkers.
C   Relies on the observation that average alcohol consumption is negatively correlated with the proportion of the population who are heavy drinkers.
D   Suggests that alcohol prevention strategies should focus on an average reduction in consumption across the population.
E   Reveals that prohibition is unsuccessful in reducing alcohol misuse.

12.2   Health promotion strategies to prevent illicit drug misuse include:
A   Use of sniffer dogs by Customs and Excise.
B   Enhancing decision-making skills in the context of antidrug norms.
C   Harm minimisation of secondary prevention.
D   Prohibition.
E   Providing alternatives to drug use through youth and community participation.

12.3   The following are regional differences in drinking behaviour across the UK:
A   The highest proportion of abstainers is in Wales.
B   The highest weekly consumption is found in Scotland.
C   Mean consumption is lowest in Northern Ireland.
D   In North East England drinking is concentrated into fewer days of the week compared to other regions.
E   The lowest proportion of heavy drinkers is in East Anglia.

(Answers overleaf)

12.1 A False The larger population of moderate/light drinkers contribute more to alcohol-related harm at a community level.
        B True See A above.
        C False Average consumption and the proportion of heavy drinkers are strongly and positively correlated.
        D True
        E False Prohibition is a separate, effective but unpopular strategy.

(Further details can be found in the *Companion to Psychiatric Studies*, p. 330.)

12.2 A False This is reducing availability.
        B True This is a resistance strategy which may reduce experimentation.
        C True
        D False This is also reducing availability.
        E True

(Further details can be found in the *Companion to Psychiatric Studies*, p. 333.)

12.3 A False The highest proportion of abstainers is in Northern Ireland.
        B False The highest weekly consumption is found in the north of England.
        C False Consumption is similar in all the home countries.
        D False This is true of Scotland.
        E False See the answer to C above.

(Further details can be found in the *Companion to Psychiatric Studies*, p. 334.)

12.4 **Alcohol problems:**
A   Are found in 10–20% of male admissions to general hospitals.
B   Account for 20% of psychiatric first admissions.
C   Occur at a rate of about 5% in the general male population.
D   Occur at a rate of about 2% in the general female population.
E   Are less common in British African Caribbean men compared to British Caucasian men.

12.5 **The natural history of alcohol dependency reveals:**
A   Relatively low rates of alcohol dependency above the age of 50.
B   That changes in the prevalence of alcohol dependency can be accounted for by mortality rates.
C   That changes in the prevalence of alcohol dependency can be accounted for by the intervention of successful treatments.
D   That once someone has had an alcohol dependency then alcohol problems will persist for life.
E   That in men, an alcohol consumption of more than 30 units per week is associated with a 350% increase in mortality rate at 15 years.

12.6 **The natural history of heroin addiction reveals that:**
A   The majority of non-regular drug users become regular drug users.
B   The majority of heroin injectors were former smokers of heroin.
C   Women who smoke heroin are less likely than men to progress to injecting heroin.
D   The excess mortality ratio for heroin addicts is approximately 20.
E   Amongst heroin addicts, mortality is higher in men compared to women.

12.7 **Edwards and Gross' alcohol dependence syndrome:**
A   Is utilised by ICD-10.
B   Includes the subjective observation that one should cut down one's level of drinking.
C   Includes alcohol withdrawal sweats.
D   Includes craving.
E   Includes subjective feelings that others are criticising one's level of drinking.

(Answers overleaf)

12.4   A   **False**   Alcohol problems are found in 20–30% of all male admissions.

       B   **True**

       C   **True**

       D   **True**

       E   **True**

(Further details can be found in the *Companion to Psychiatric Studies*, p. 335.)

12.5   A   **True**

       B   **False**   Rather, people move in and out of problem drinking.

       C   **False**   See B above.

       D   **False**   See B above.

       E   **True**   These results are from a longitudinal study of Swedish conscripts.

(Further details can be found in the *Companion to Psychiatric Studies*, p. 337.)

12.6   A   **False**

       B   **True**   Although the majority of smokers do not move to injecting.

       C   **True**

       D   **False**   The excess mortality ratio is 12, i.e. about 2% annually.

       E   **False**   There is no sex difference.

(Further details can be found in the *Companion to Psychiatric Studies*, p. 337.)

12.7   A.   **True**

       B   **False**   This is a CAGE question.

       C   **True**

       D   **True**

       E   **False**   This is another CAGE question.

(Further details can be found in the *Companion to Psychiatric Studies*, p. 338.)

12.8   People with mental illness who also take illicit drugs:

A   Do so at a rate of between 20 and 50%.

B   Have more frequent relapses compared to those with mental illness who do not take illicit drugs.

C   Have more severe relapses compared to those with mental illness who do not take illicit drugs.

D   Have more episodes of hospitalisation compared to those with mental illness who do not take illicit drugs.

E   Are several times more violent towards others compared to those with mental illness who do not take illicit drugs.

12.9   Features of Cloninger's type 1 male alcoholics include:

A   Social detachment.

B   Distractibility.

C   Early onset.

D   Severe social problems.

E   Similarity of the drinking pattern to the biological father.

12.10   Women with alcohol dependency syndrome:

A   Make up 20% of the total number of people with alcohol problems seen in psychiatric practice.

B   Particularly attribute the onset of their drinking problems to stress as compared to men.

C   Compared to men, more commonly develop an alcohol problem after adverse life events.

D   When compared to men, are particularly prone to depression.

E   Are more likely to have experienced childhood sexual abuse.

12.11   The genetics of alcohol misuse has revealed:

A   Little difference in the concordance of monozygotic twins compared to dizygotic twins.

B   Higher levels of alcohol dehydrogenase in the Oriental population.

C   A genetic basis for the problems in cognitive abstraction found in those with alcohol dependency.

D   Greater distractibility in the children of people with alcohol dependency.

E   A genetic basis for the problem in planning memory found in those with alcohol dependency.

(Answers overleaf)

12.8 A True
      B True
      C True
      D True
      E True

(Further details can be found in the *Companion to Psychiatric Studies*, pp. 338–389.)

12.9 A False
      B False
      C False
      D False
      E False

The features listed in the question are all those of Cloninger's type 2 alcoholism. (Further details can be found in the *Companion to Psychiatric Studies*, p. 339.)

12.10 A False The proportion is one-third.
       B True
       C False Adverse events do not predict alcohol problems.
       D True
       E True More female alcoholics report abuse than in the general population.

(Further details can be found in the *Companion to Psychiatric Studies*, p. 340.)

12.11 A False There is greater concordance in drinking style in monozygotic twins.
       B False Orientals tend to have low levels of acetaldehyde dehydrogenase.
       C False There may, however, be greater problems with abstraction in the children of alcoholics.
       D True
       E False See the answer to C above.

(Further details can be found in the *Companion to Psychiatric Studies*, p. 342.)

12.12 The 'carry-over' phenomenon:

A Refers to the observation that even 1 unit of alcohol may set off a psychological 'trip wire' which then reinstates a former pattern of alcohol drinking.

B Refers to the observation that even 1 unit of alcohol may set off a physiological 'trip wire' which reinstates a former pattern of alcohol drinking.

C Is also termed reinstatement.

D Has been demonstrated in monkeys and rats.

E Is the return to a former pattern of response to alcohol in former alcoholics who drink again.

12.13 Alcoholic hallucinosis:

A Is usually associated with auditory hallucinations.

B Occurs in clear consciousness.

C Persists 6 months after abstinence in only 5–10% of cases.

D Commonly goes on to fulfil diagnostic criteria for schizophrenia.

E Occurs more commonly when there is a family history of schizophrenia.

12.14 Fetal alcohol syndrome:

A Is characterised by developmental retardation.

B Is characterised by growth retardation.

C Is characterised by facial abnormalities.

D Is characterised by neurological abnormalities.

E Is exacerbated by smoking.

12.15 Regarding cannabis:

A There is no scientific evidence for the existence of cannabis dependency.

B It is associated with psychotic symptoms.

C Marijuana smoke contains the same carcinogens as tobacco.

D It is available on prescription in parts of the USA.

E There is little evidence of long-term negative consequences of chronic use.

(Answers overleaf)

12.12   A. **False**   There in no such evidence.
          B   **False**   Three drinks may be a 'physiological trip wire'.
          C   **True**
          D   **True**   It has been demonstrated in those made physically dependent.
          E   **True**

(Further details can be found in the *Companion to Psychiatric Studies*, p. 343.)

12.13   A **True**
          B **True**
          C **True**
          D **False**   Only a minority go on to show schizophrenic deterioration.
          E **False**   Such a family history is, however, associated with persistent hallucinations and deterioration.

(Further details can be found in the *Companion to Psychiatric Studies*, p. 344.)

12.14   A **True**
          B **True**
          C **True**
          D **True**
          E **True**

(Further details can be found in the *Companion to Psychiatric Studies*, p. 348.)

12.15   A **False**   It occurs in a small proportion of users.
          B **True**
          C **True**
          D **True**   It is available for symptomatic treatment in, for example, cancer.
          E **True**

(Further details can be found in the *Companion to Psychiatric Studies*, p. 360.)

13. Schizophrenia

13.1 The following psychiatrists were first to describe the terms that follow their names:
A Hecker – Katatonie.
B Morel – démence précoce.
C Kraepelin – manic-depressive insanity.
D Griesinger – schizophreniform psychosis.
E Manfred Bleuler – schizophrenia.

13.2 Eugen Bleuler described 'fundamental' features of schizophrenia, which came to be known as the 'four As'. These included:
A Loosening of associations.
B Aimlessness.
C Ambitendence.
D Autism.
F Ambivalence

13.3 The following statements are true:
A The International Pilot Study of Schizophrenia (WHO 1973) conducted research in Peru.
B In the 1950s, psychiatrists in the USA were more likely to diagnose schizophrenia than their contemporaries in the UK.
C The St. Louis criteria for schizophrenia (Feighner et al 1972) specify that delusional ideation must be present for the disorder to be diagnosed.
D ICD-10 criteria for schizophrenia require a minimum illness duration of 6 months.
E It is difficult for acute first episode cases to fulfil DSM-IV criteria for schizophrenia.

13.4 The following statements about the phenomenology of schizophrenia are correct:
A Hallucinations may occur in all modalities.
B Delusional mood is a mood change secondary to a delusional belief.
C Pseudohallucinations occur in patients with schizophrenia.
D While incongruity of affect is a not uncommon sign, it may also be a symptom.
E Automatism is a feature of catatonic schizophrenia.

(Answers overleaf)

13.1 A **False** Hecker described Hebephrenie 3 years after Kahlbaum first described Katatonie in 1868.
  B **True** Morel described démence précoce in 1856.
  C **True** Kraepelin described manic-depressive insanity in 1896.
  D **False** Schizophreniform psychosis was first described by Langfeldt.
  E **False** Eugen Bleuler first described schizophrenia, in 1911.

(Further details can be found in the *Companion to Psychiatric Studies*, pp. 369–370.)

13.2 A **True**
  B **False** The 'four As' included disorders of affect.
  C **False** Ambitendence is a catatonic phenomenon.
  D **True**
  E **True**

(Further details can be found in the *Companion to Psychiatric Studies*, pp. 369–370.)

13.3 A **False** Colombia was the only South American country involved in this study.
  B **True** US psychiatrists made the diagnosis twice as commonly.
  C **False** The Feighner criteria are the only currently used criteria that do not specify particular kinds of delusion.
  D **False** The duration criterion in ICD-10 is 1 month.
  E **True** DSM-IV require a 6-month symptom duration.

(Further details can be found in the *Companion to Psychiatric Studies*, pp. 371–372.)

13.4 A **True**
  B **False** Delusional mood precedes frank delusions.
  C **True**
  D **True**
  E **False** Automatisms are usually associated with epilepsy (see *Companion to Psychiatric Studies*, p. 317).

(Further details can be found in the *Companion to Psychiatric Studies*, pp. 373–374.)

13.5 **The symptoms of schizophrenia have been classed as positive and negative, and later grouped into two and then three syndromes; with regard to these distinctions, the following statements are true:**

A Hughlings Jackson introduced the terms positive and negative symptoms in relation to schizophrenia.

B Crow included hallucinations among the features of type I syndrome.

C The position of thought disorder is clearly specified in Crow's typology.

D Crow's type II syndrome has much in common with Liddle's psychomotor poverty.

E On PET scanning, patterns of metabolism are different in psychomotor poverty and reality distortion.

13.6 **Thought disorder in schizophrenia:**

A Occurs in the majority.

B Is characterised by a high 'type : token ratio'.

C Was first described by Kelly.

D Is diagnostically useful.

E May be indicated by clanging.

13.7 **Kraepelin originally described three varieties of schizophrenia. Other varieties and related conditions were later added by others, as shown below:**

A Simple schizophrenia – Manfred Bleuler.

B Schizoaffective psychosis – Kasanin.

C Postschizophrenic depression – Andreasson.

D Overt schizophrenia – Eugen Bleuler.

E Schizotypal disorder – Kenneth Kendler.

13.8 **The following statements regarding the epidemiology of schizophrenia are true:**

A The worldwide annual incidence is approximately 15 cases per 100 000 per annum.

B The paranoid form of the illness has become less common in Northern Europe during the course of the 20th century.

C The age of onset is generally earlier in females than in males.

D It is clearly established that the incidence of schizophrenia is increased in migrants.

E There is a positive association between schizophrenia and rheumatoid arthritis.

(Answers overleaf)

13.5   A   False
          B   True
          C   False
          D   True
          E   True

(Further details can be found in the *Companion to Psychiatric Studies*, p. 375.)

13.6   A   False   Thought disorder is rare.
          B   False   Schizophrenics tend to have a low type:token ratio, i.e. they have a restricted range of words.
          C   False   Kelly described personal construct theory.
          D   False   Thought disorder can be found in mania and in highly regarded literature.
          E   True   Clang association links words by sound rather than meaning (see *Companion to Psychiatric Studies*, p. 251).

(Further details can be found in the *Companion to Psychiatric Studies*, pp. 376–377.)

13.7   A   False
          B   True   Kasanin published his work in 1933.
          C   False
          D   False
          E   True

(Further details can be found in the *Companion to Psychiatric Studies*, p. 377.)

13.8   A   True
          B   False   Hebephrenic and catatonic forms have become less common; paranoid more common.
          C   False   Onset in males is generally 4–5 years earlier.
          D   False   It is more often diagnosed in migrants but this does not necessarily mean that the incidence is greater.
          E   False   There is a negative association between schizophrenia and rheumatoid arthritis.

(Further details can be found in the *Companion to Psychiatric Studies*, pp. 378–380.)

13.9 **Regarding biological factors in the aetiology of schizophrenia:**

A Adoption studies have shown that children who are adopted away from biological mothers with schizophrenia have the same rates of schizophrenia as the normal population.

B A relative excess of people born in January develop schizophrenia.

C Subtle cytoarchitectural changes of the caudate nucleus are common in schizophrenia.

D The brains of people with schizophrenia are lighter than normal controls.

E Recent studies indicate that the connectivity between cerebral areas is disturbed in schizophrenia.

13.10 **Regarding social factors in the aetiology of schizophrenia:**

A The term 'schizophrenogenic' mother was introduced in the 1960s.

B Lidz described 'marital schism'.

C Bateson described the 'double-bind hypothesis'.

D People who develop schizophrenia experience significantly more life events in the 12 weeks prior to the first onset of their illness than controls.

E If a person with newly diagnosed schizophrenia is discharged to live with a high 'expressed emotion' relative, with whom they have face-to-face contact for more than 35 hours per week, the chance of relapse at 1 year is less than 30%.

13.11 **Regarding psychological theories of schizophrenia, the following are true:**

A Meta-representation is a form of complex hallucinatory experience in which the patients perceives entire environments.

B The cognitive process postulated to underlie delusions of passivity is an inability to monitor willed action.

C Poverty of action is said to be due to an inability to generate willed action.

D Delusions of persecution may be understood as a result of the inability to infer the intentions of others.

E Latent inhibition refers to the phenomenon whereby repeated exposure to a stimulus without consequence speeds up subsequent conditioning to that stimulus.

(Answers overleaf)

13.9 **A** **False** Children with an affected parent have an increased risk of schizophrenia.
B **True** Winter birth is associated with the later development of schizophrenia.
C **False** Such subtle changes have been described in the hippocampus.
D **True**
E **True**

(Further details can be found in the *Companion to Psychiatric Studies*, pp. 381–382.)

13.10 **A** **False** Freda Fromm-Reichmann coined the phrase in the 1940s.
B **True** See Lidz et al 1965.
C **True** See Bateson et al 1956.
D **False** Brown and Birley, in an article published in 1968, identified an increase in life events in the 3 weeks prior to onset.
E **False** The relapse rate is about 50%.

(Further details can be found in the *Companion to Psychiatric Studies*, pp. 382–384.)

13.11 **A** **False** Meta-representation is the mechanism which enables us to be aware of our goals and intentions and infer those of others.
B **True**
C **True**
D **True**
E **False** It retards subsequent conditioning to the stimulus.

(Further details can be found in the *Companion to Psychiatric Studies*, pp. 384–385.)

13.12 **A relatively good outcome has been said to occur in schizophrenia:**

A When the onset is acute.

B In women rather than men.

C Where schizoid traits were present premorbidly.

D In industrialised rather than in underdeveloped countries.

E Where there is a positive family history of depressive illness.

13.13 **The following statements are true:**

A Between 1950 and 1990 the number of available mental hospital beds in most industrialised countries fell by at least 50%.

B The outcome of schizophrenia, in terms of relapse rates, is better in Czechoslovakia than in Colombia.

C The onset of schizophrenia is more likely to be acute and sudden in developing rather than developed countries.

D People with schizophrenia in rural Scotland have a lower level of overall functioning relative to comparable people with schizophrenia in urban South London.

E The prognosis of schizophrenia in industrial countries is better now than 100 years ago.

13.14 **The following statements are true regarding the treatment of schizophrenia:**

A The expected relapse rate at 2 years is the same with either conventional oral or depot antipsychotic therapy.

B There is overwhelming evidence to suggest that negative symptoms of schizophrenia are reduced by conventional oral antipsychotics.

C It is good practice to routinely prescribe an anticholinergic drug alongside an antipsychotic.

D Involuntary spontaneous disorders of movement can occur in people with schizophrenia who are antipsychotic naïve.

E Psychodynamic psychotherapy may be of some value in the acute stage of the illness.

(Answers overleaf)

13.12 A True
 B True
 C False
 D False
 E True

(Further details can be found in the *Companion to Psychiatric Studies*, pp. 385–386.)

13.13 A True
 B False Schizophrenia has a better outcome in underdeveloped countries.
 C True This was a finding of the Determinants of Outcome study.
 D False Rural populations tend to have a better outcome.
 E True This is due to better treatment and/or a change in the nature of the disease.

(Further details can be found in the *Companion to Psychiatric Studies*, pp. 385–387.)

13.14 A True
 B False The trials are conflicting.
 C False Anticholinergics may not work, may worsen symptoms, may increase tardive dyskinesia and have abuse potential.
 D True See, for example, Owens et al 1982.
 E False Psychodynamic psychotherapy prolongs hospital treatment.

(Further details can be found in the *Companion to Psychiatric Studies*, pp. 388–390.)

14. Mood disorder

14.1 **To meet the DSM-IV criteria for major depressive episode:**
  A   There must be a loss of interest or pleasure.
  B   There must be disturbance of sleep.
  C   Symptoms secondary to general medical conditions can be included.
  D   Symptoms must be present for a minimum of 2 weeks.
  E   Weight loss can be considered but not weight gain.

14.2 **In atypical depression:**
  A   Increase in food intake and sleeping is common.
  B   Mood is unreactive.
  C   Personality issues are prominent.
  D   It is claimed that tricyclic antidepressants are more effective than monoamine oxidase inhibitors (MAOIs).
  E   Sensitivity to personal rejection is a feature.

14.3 **Brief recurrent depression:**
  A   Has a recognised comorbidity with major depression.
  B   Is not classed as a separate entity in ICD-10.
  C   Generally responds well to tricyclic antidepressants.
  D   Is associated with anxiety.
  E   Rarely leads to deliberate self-harm.

14.4 **Mania:**
  A   Is characterised by disinhibition of psychomotor function.
  B   Can include mixed state symptoms in DSM-IV.
  C   Can be usefully divided into psychotic and non-psychotic mania.
  D   Can be diagnosed with DSM-IV if elevated mood is present for 1 week.
  E   Excludes symptoms due to drugs or medical conditions in DSM-IV.

(Answers overleaf)   **111**

14.1 A True
       B False
       C False
       D True
       E False

Five or more of a number of symptoms must be present for a period of 2 weeks and represent a change in functioning. At least one of the symptoms must be (1) depressed mood or (2) loss of interest or pleasure. Symptoms secondary to medical conditions are excluded. (Further details can be found in the *Companion to Psychiatric Studies*, pp. 400–401 (including Table 14.1).)

14.2 A True
       B False Mood is unusually reactive.
       C True
       D False MAOIs are more effective.
       E True

(Further details can be found in the *Companion to Psychiatric Studies*, p. 405.)

14.3 A True   There is a striking comorbidity with major depression and dysthymia. Patients may show conversion from major depression to brief recurrent depression and vice versa.
       B False It is F38.10 in ICD-10, but is not in DSM-IV.
       C False Treatment trials have been disappointing.
       D True   There may be important associations with short periods of anxiety and with the risk of deliberate self-harm.
       E False See D above.

(Further details can be found in the *Companion to Psychiatric Studies*, p. 405.)

14.4 A True
       B False DSM-IV has a separate category for mixed episode.
       C False This distinction is arbitrary.
       D True
       E True

(Further details can be found in the *Companion to Psychiatric Studies*, p. 406 (including Table 14.4).)

14.5   **Seasonal affective disorder (SAD):**
   A   Was first described in surveys of the general population.
   B   Includes sensitivity to rejection as a symptom.
   C   Commonly presents with hypersomnia and hyperphagia.
   D   Is best treated with bright light therapy in the early morning.
   E   Is associated with an increased sensitivity to light in the suppression of melatonin.

14.6   **The following statements are true of the epidemiology of bipolar affective disorder:**
   A   Lifetime rates are higher than those for unipolar disorder.
   B   The sex ratio is equal.
   C   The age of onset is usually earlier than in unipolar disorder.
   D   Females have a higher proportion of manic episodes.
   E   Bipolar II is often misclassified as unipolar depression.

14.7   **Concerning the genetic epidemiology of depression:**
   A   Over 50% of genetic liability to major depression is shared with the personality trait neuroticism.
   B   The best predictors of a subsequent depressive episode include stressful life events and high neuroticism but exclude genetic factors.
   C   Genetic factors account for > 90% of the variance in liability to depression.
   D   The Australian Twin Register Study showed a clear genetic pattern to the inheritance of neuroticism.
   E   The Australian Twin Register Study found that lability in neuroticism was primarily affected by adverse life events.

(Answers overleaf)

14.5 A **False** SAD was first described in subjects who answered newspaper advertisements.

B **False** Those with SAD describe features of atypical depression – hypersomnia, hyperphagia, tiredness and low mood in winter but do not show rejection sensitivity.

C **True** See B above.

D **False** The status of SAD and light therapy remains unclear and patients with winter episodes of depression are best treated conventionally.

E **False** It has been difficult to show any benefit in SAD of bright over dim light or increased sensitivity to light in the suppression of melatonin.

(Further details can be found in the *Companion to Psychiatric Studies*, p. 407.)

14.6 A **False** The rates are 0.3–1.5% and 1.5–19% respectively.

B **True**

C **True**

D **False** Women have fewer manic episodes.

E **True**

(Further details can be found in the *Companion to Psychiatric Studies*, p. 409.)

14.7 A **True** Of the genetic liability to depression, 55% appears to be shared with the personality trait neuroticism.

B **False** Kendler's group developed an exploratory model which accounted for 50% of the variance in liability to major depression over 1 year – stressful life events, genetic factors, a previous depressive episode and neuroticism emerged as the best predictors.

C **False** See B above.

D **True** The Australian Twin Register Study showed a substantial genetic involvement in the average level of neuroticism and current symptoms.

E **True** Neither genes nor shared environment was a significant cause of lability which was primarily affected by adverse life events.

(Further details can be found in the *Companion to Psychiatric Studies*, p. 410.)

14.8 **Regarding environmental risk factors for affective disorders:**

A   Kendler's studies show life events as strong predictors of the onset of major depression.

B   Genetically controlled studies have shown the importance of threat/loss events.

C   Brown's studies have shown that life events have a crucial role in recurrent episodes of major depression.

D   Kendler showed that genetic liability to major depression was associated with increased risk of encountering adversity.

E   Over 50% of the genetic liability to depression may be mediated by genetically determined life events.

14.9 **Evidence for an environmental component of the aetiology of bipolar disorder comes from:**

A   Studies suggesting there is a significant excess of life events prior to the onset of bipolar disorder.

B   1 in 2000 mothers developing a manic psychosis following childbirth.

C   Bipolar depression being more common in the Autumn.

D   Mania being more common in the Summer.

E   Individual seasonality effects on bipolar disorder being present in 50% of patients.

(Answers overleaf)

14.8 A True
       B True   The differential effects of threat and loss have been clarified by genetically controlled studies.
       C False
       D True   Kendler's community studies found that genetic liability to major depression was associated with a significantly increased risk of assault, serious marital problems, divorce/break-up, job loss, serious illness, major financial problems and problems with relatives/friends.
       E False About 10% of the total genetic liability to major depression may be mediated by genetically determined life events.

(Further details can be found in the *Companion to Psychiatric Studies*, pp. 412–413.)

14.9 A False Effects of life events on onset/recurrence of bipolar disorder have received much less attention than for non-endogenous major depression, although there may be a small excess of life events in advance of manic recurrence in bipolar illness.
       B False 1 in 500 mothers may develop a psychosis within 3 weeks of childbirth and this is usually manic in form.
       C True   Mania appears to have no seasonal variation but bipolar depression may be more common in the Autumn.
       D False See C above.
       E False Around 10% of patients seem to manifest individual seasonality which may be useful in advising on self-management.

(Further details can be found in the *Companion to Psychiatric Studies*, p. 413.)

14.10   Tryptophan depletion:

A   Results in depressed mood in males with a positive family history of depression.

B   Produces a distinct relapse in recovered depressives treated with selective serotonin reuptake inhibitors (SSRIs).

C   Induced depressive symptoms tend to be atypical.

D   Induces suicidal thoughts of greater severity on their return.

E   Suggests a link between neurotransmitter function and symptoms that may explain the need for long-term antidepressant treatment in the vulnerable.

14.11   Sleep disturbance in affective disorder:

A   Is most typically manifest as early morning wakening in depression.

B   Can be used as a treatment in depression.

C   Is associated with increased rapid eye movement (REM) sleep latency in depression.

D   Is associated with a reduced total length of slow wave sleep in depression.

E   May be cholinergically driven.

(Answers overleaf)

14.10 **A** **True** Tryptophan depletion produces reductions in mood in females and males with a family history of depression.

B **True** It is striking that in patients who have recovered from a depressive episode with SSRI, tryptophan depletion produces a transient but clear-cut return of severe symptoms.

C **False** The prominent objective symptoms of retardation and cognitive distortion return in a stereotyped and severe way.

D **False** By contrast, suicidal thoughts and other cognitive measures do not.

E **True** The apparent immediacy of the link between neurotransmitter function and symptoms may be why vulnerable groups need long-term treatment with antidepressants to remain well.

(Further details can be found in the *Companion to Psychiatric Studies*, p. 416.)

14.11 **A** **True** Early morning wakening is the most typical form of sleep disturbance in depression, but not the only pattern.

B **True** Patients with depression can respond to sleep deprivation with a transient improvement in mood.

C **False** The most characteristic sleep EEG patterns in melancholia are decrease in total length of slow wave sleep and shortened latency to the appearance of REM sleep.

D **False** See C above.

E **True** It has been suggested that REM induction represents a cholinergic mechanism that may become abnormal in depression.

(Further details can be found in the *Companion to Psychiatric Studies*, p. 418.)

14.12   **Treatment with selective serotonin reuptake inhibitors (SSRIs):**
   A   Can result in orgasmic impotence.
   B   Is associated with nausea and vomiting that diminishes with time.
   C   Is associated with sleep disturbance.
   D   Has replaced that with tricyclics as the treatment of choice for depression.
   E   Has simple dosing regimes.

14.13   **Treatment with electroconvulsive therapy (ECT):**
   A   Is indicated for depression with psychotic features.
   B   Is more effective if given bilaterally.
   C   Can be used following failure of response to pharmacotherapy.
   D   Usually requires between 10 and 12 applications.
   E   Under naturalistic conditions, is associated with a 50% response rate.

14.14   **In combination treatment of depression:**
   A   Lithium augmentation of antidepressants has an acute effect in 50% of refractory depressed patients.
   B   The combination of tryptophan and clomipramine is contraindicated because of the enhanced serotonergic effect.
   C   Relapse of depressive symptoms has been shown on withdrawal of L-tryptophan.
   D   There is no evidence to support thyroid augmentation.
   E   Tri-iodothyronine (T_3) is the thyroid preparation used for augmentation purposes.

(Answers overleaf)

14.12 **A** **True** SSRIs can cause orgasmic impotence which can be a major problem in long-term use, or a possible advantage in those with premature ejaculation.

       B **True** The nausea and vomiting associated with SSRIs tends to diminish with time.

       C **True**

       D **False** SSRIs have not replaced tricyclics but appear to be prescribed in addition to them.

       E **True** SSRIs are easier to prescribe because of simpler dosing regimes.

(Further details can be found in the *Companion to Psychiatric Studies*, p. 419.)

14.13 **A** **True** The indications for ECT are usually psychotic or severe endogenous depression and failure of drug treatment.

       B **True** Unless contraindicated by confusion, bilateral ECT is preferable.

       C **True** See A above.

       D **False** The number of treatments varies but is usually between four and six.

       E **False** The earliest changes occur in feeding and locomotion and the response rate under naturalistic conditions is around 80%.

(Further details can be found in the *Companion to Psychiatric Studies*, p. 420.)

14.14 **A** **True** Lithium augmentation to tricyclic antidepressants, SSRIs or MAOIs appears to be associated with an acute antidepressant effect in up to 50% of refractory patients.

       B **False** The combination of tryptophan and clomipramine is not contraindicated.

       C **True** The withdrawal of tryptophan produces relapse in patients treated long-term with combination treatment.

       D **False** There is evidence to support augmentation of antidepressants with tri-iodothyronine.

       E **True**

(Further details can be found in the *Companion to Psychiatric Studies*, pp. 420–421.)

14.15 **The following statements are true of the treatment of mania:**

    A   Lithium is ineffective in acute mania.

    B   Sodium valproate may be the drug of choice for rapid cycling bipolar disorder.

    C   Electroconvulsive therapy (ECT) is effective in refractory mania.

    D   A high therapeutic index is the reason for plasma monitoring of lithium levels.

    E   The most common side-effects of lithium are fine tremor, polyuria and weight gain.

(Answers overleaf)

14.15 A **False** Lithium itself is effective in acute mania.
B **True** Valproate may be the preferred choice when rapid cycling or mixed states are prominent.
C **True** ECT has been used effectively in refractory mania.
D **False** Lithium has an unusually low therapeutic index.
E **True** The most common side-effects of lithium are fine tremor, polyuria and weight gain.

(Further details can be found in the *Companion to Psychiatric Studies*, pp. 422–423.)

15. Paranoid disorders

15.1 **As defined by ICD-10 or DSM-IV, persistent delusional disorders:**
A   Are commonly diagnosed in clinical practice.
B   May present with bizarre delusions.
C   May be secondary to alcohol abuse.
D   Are usually associated with a severe disturbance of social functioning.
E   Can be secondary to organic disorders.

15.2 **The following statements are true of persistent delusional disorders as defined by ICD-10 or DSM-IV:**
A   Delusional disorder has a clear genetic basis.
B   Relatives of people with delusional disorders are more likely to show evidence of psychopathology than the generality of the normal population.
C   The prevalence of schizophrenia is the same in first- and second-degree relatives of patients with delusional disorder as it is in the first and second relatives of patients with schizophrenia.
D   People who later develop delusional disorder have been described as having avoidant or sensitive premorbid personalities.
E   Delusional disorder is less common in migrants.

15.3 **The following are recognised potential risk factors for the development of delusional disorder:**
A   Imprisonment.
B   Deafness.
C   Amputation of a limb.
D   Gynaecological surgery.
E   Previous history of psoriasis.

15.4 **Regarding the epidemiology of delusional disorder:**
A   It typically presents before the age of 30.
B   Males are more commonly affected than females.
C   It is commoner amongst lower socioeconomic groups.
D   The incidence is 30 per 100 000.
E   The prevalence is 1–3 per 100 000 per year.

(Answers overleaf)

15.1 A **False** Delusional disorders are rare.
B **False** The delusions are non-bizarre.
C **False** The absence of substance misuse is a defined characteristic.
D **False** Preserved social functioning is a defined characteristic.
E **False** The absence of organic brain disease is a defined characteristic.

(Further details can be found in the *Companion to Psychiatric Studies*, p. 432.)

15.2 A **False** The disorder is associated with a general but non-specific psychopathology in family members.
B **True** See A above.
C **False** The rate of schizophrenia is not increased in family members.
D **True**
E **False** It may be more common in migrants.

(Further details can be found in the *Companion to Psychiatric Studies*, p. 433.)

15.3 A **True** Isolation of any kind may precipitate paranoid delusions.
B **True**
C **False**
D **False**
E **False**

(Further details can be found in the *Companion to Psychiatric Studies*, p. 434.)

15.4 A **False** The typical presentation is in middle or old age.
B **False** The sex ratio is equal.
C **True**
D **False** This is the prevalence.
E **False** This is the incidence.

(Further details can be found in the *Companion to Psychiatric Studies*, p. 434.)

15.5 **The following are good prognostic indicators for delusional disorder:**

A Divorced.
B Employed.
C Instigation of treatment within 6 months of onset.
D Lack of clear precipitants.
E Jealous subtype.

15.6 **Regarding morbid jealousy:**

A It is also known as Othello syndrome.
B It may be a symptom of alcohol dependence.
C It may be associated with serious threat of violence.
D It occurs in both men and women.
E Geographical separation of the patient and suspected individual (victim) should be avoided if possible, as it is likely to make the situation worse.

15.7 **Monosymptomatic hypochondriacal psychosis:**

A May be characterised by a delusion of extreme halitosis.
B May be characterised by a delusion of infestation.
C Is usually associated with disintegration of the personality.
D Usually has a sudden onset.
E Is associated with a past history of abnormal personality or substance misuse.

15.8 **Dysmorphophobia:**

A Is also known as body dysmorphic disorder.
B Is usually associated with adolescent onset.
C Sufferers rarely have a past history of surgical procedures.
D May be associated with obsessive–compulsive disorder.
E Responds better to selective serotonin reuptake inhibitors (SSRIs) than to neuroleptic treatment.

15.9 **The following statements are true:**

A Cotard described délire de négation.
B Almost all people with Cotard's syndrome have depressive symptoms.
C Typically Othello syndrome occurs before the age of 40.
D Geographical separation of patient and victim augments delusional jealousy.
E In morbid jealousy, psychotic individuals have a better prognosis than those with neurosis.

(Answers overleaf)

15.5   A   **False**   Being married is associated with a better prognosis.
        B   **True**
        C   **True**
        D   **False**   Reactive delusional disorder has a better prognosis.
        E   **True**

(Further details can be found in the *Companion to Psychiatric Studies*, p. 434.)

15.6   A   **True**
        B   **True**
        C   **True**
        D   **True**
        E   **False**

(Further details can be found in the *Companion to Psychiatric Studies*, pp. 438–439.)

15.7   A   **True**
        B   **True**
        C   **False**   Personality is preserved.
        D   **False**   The onset is usually insidious.
        E   **True**

(Further details can be found in the *Companion to Psychiatric Studies*, p. 437.)

15.8   A   **True**
        B   **True**
        C   **False**   Patients commonly seek and sometimes receive surgery.
        D   **True**
        E   **True**   See McElroy et al 1993.

(Further details can be found in the *Companion to Psychiatric Studies*, p. 437.)

15.9   A   **True**
        B   **True**   About 90% have depressive symptoms.
        C   **False**   Onset is typically after the age of 40.
        D   **False**   Separation can reduce symptom intensity.
        E   **True**

(Further details can be found in the *Companion to Psychiatric Studies*, pp. 438–439.)

15.10   **Erotomania:**
A   Occurs in mania.
B   Is commoner in men.
C   Has been construed as a manifestation of unmet narcissistic needs.
D   May be associated with a history of antisocial behaviour.
E   Was described by de Clérambault in 1842.

15.11   **The following are found in the Ganser syndrome:**
A   Apathy.
B   Vorbeireden.
C   Disorientation.
D   Hallucinations.
E   Anxiety.

15.12   **In folie à deux:**
A   The recipient usually has a lower IQ than the dominant partner.
B   The dominant partner has been postulated to have repressed oedipal fantasies.
C   The dominant partner is more likely to be male.
D   Comorbid learning disability is common.
E   Hallucinations frequently occur.

(Answers overleaf)

15.10 **A** **True**
       B **False**   It is more common in women.
       C **True**   See, for example, Segal 1989.
       D **True**
       E **False**   It was described by de Clérambault in 1942.

(Further details can be found in the *Companion to Psychiatric Studies*, p. 439.)

15.11 **A** **True**
       B **True**   Vorbeireden is the giving of approximate answers.
       C **True**
       D **True**
       E **True**

(Further details can be found in the *Companion to Psychiatric Studies*, p. 443.)

15.12 **A** **True**
       B **False**   These have been described in the passive acceptor.
       C **False**   The sex ratio is equal.
       D **True**
       E **True**

(Further details can be found in the *Companion to Psychiatric Studies*, pp. 443–444.)

16. Neuroimaging

16.1   X-ray computerised tomography (CT):

A   Enables a three-dimensional image to be constructed.
B   Uses more radiation than a [^{99m}Tc]HMPAO SPECT scan.
C   May be useful in the diagnosis of Binswanger's disease.
D   Studies were the first to demonstrate ventricular dilatation in schizophrenia.
E   Enables hippocampal thickness to be measured.

16.2   Magnetic resonance imaging (MRI):

A   Depends on three-dimensional magnetic field gradients for spatial encoding.
B   Uses the precession of atomic nuclei.
C   Depends upon the Larmor frequency.
D   May utilise the T_1* phenomenon.
E   May use a spin–echo configuration.

16.3   Magnetic resonance spectroscopy (MRS):

A   Enables the measurement of the concentration of different molecular groups.
B   Is a method of analytical chemistry in vitro.
C   Commonly uses ^{31}P in vivo.
D   Uses ^{7}Li for in vivo lithium measurement in the brain.
E   Can use ^{1}H as an in vivo measure of creatinine.

16.4   Functional magnetic resonance imaging (fMRI):

A   May use fast low-angle shot (FLASH) radiofrequency pulses.
B   May use echo-planar imaging (EPI) to reduce scanning time.
C   Enables the study of brain functions in the 1–10 second range.
D   Using paramagnetic agents enables regional blood volumes to be computed.
E   Uses the BOLD (blood oxygen level dependent) phenomenon as the commonest fMRI method.

(Answers overleaf)

16.1   A   **True**   Provided there is sufficient computer power.
           B   **False**   The radiation dose for X-ray CT is 1.8 mSv; for a [^{99m}Tc]HMPAO SPECT scan it is 4.7 mSv.
           C   **True**   It can detect white matter translucencies.
           D   **False**   CT studies confirmed suggestions of pneumo-encephalographic studies.
           E   **True**   It is done by scanning along the longitudinal axis of the temporal lobes.

(Further details can be found in the *Companion to Psychiatric Studies*, pp. 447–448.)

16.2   A   **True**
           B   **True**
           C   **True**
           D   **False** T_1 and T_2* relaxation times are relevant.
           E   **True**   It is used to enhance the signal by reducing field inhomogeneities.

(Further details can be found in the *Companion to Psychiatric Studies*, p. 448.)

16.3   A   **True**   It is possible because they have different resonance frequencies.
           B   **True**
           C   **True**
           D   **True**
           E   **True**   See *Companion to Psychiatric Studies*, Figure 16.2 (p. 449).

(Further details can be found in the *Companion to Psychiatric Studies*, p. 449.)

16.4   A   **True**   It is done to reduce imaging time.
           B   **True**   EPI is even quicker than FLASH.
           C   **False**   Brain functions can be studies in the 100 ms to 1 second range.
           D   **True**
           E   **True**

(Further details can be found in the *Companion to Psychiatric Studies*, pp. 449–450.)

16.5 **The following statements regarding functional magnetic resonance imaging (fMRI) are true:**

A The signal-to-noise ratio varies inversely with the strength of the static magnetic field.

B Most published studies use a field strength < 1.5 tesla.

C The relative importance of the haematocrit is negligible.

D The (blood oxygen level dependent) BOLD signal comes mostly from the venous system.

E Spin–echo sequences may be used for signal extraction from smaller blood vessels.

16.6 **The following techniques have demonstrated the associated findings:**

A Structural MRI – reduction of temporal lobe volume in schizophrenia.

B MRS – temporal lobe increase in phosphomonoesters in schizophrenia.

C MRS – demonstration of respiratory alkalosis during a panic attack.

D fMRI – amygdala activation on emotional stimulation.

E fMRI – activation of the insular cortex in obsessive–compulsive disorder during an anxiety-provoking condition.

16.7 **The following statements are true:**

A Ingvar and Franzén originally described hyperfrontality in schizophrenia.

B Neuroleptic medication increases basal ganglia metabolism.

C Recent brain imaging studies have sought to examine the functional anatomy of hallucinations.

D Depressed subjects show basal ganglia overactivity on single photon emission tomography (SPECT).

E Subjects with obsessional disorder consistently show evidence of symptom-related paralimbic overactivity on SPECT.

(Answers overleaf)

16.5   **A**   **False**   The signal relatively increases and the noise decreases in stronger fields.
     B   **False**   Most use 1.5 tesla or more.
     C   **False**   The haematocrit contribution is unknown.
     D   **True**
     E   **True**

(Further details can be found in the *Companion to Psychiatric Studies*, p. 450.)

16.6   **A**   **True**
     B   **False**   Phosphomonoesters are decreased; diesters are increased.
     C   **True**   Respiratory alkalosis can be demonstrated during hyperventilation.
     D   **True**
     E   **True**

(Further details can be found in the *Companion to Psychiatric Studies*, pp. 450–451.)

16.7   **A**   **False**   They described hypofrontality.
     B   **True**
     C   **True**   See, for example, McGuire et al 1995.
     D   **False**   The basal ganglia are underactive in depression.
     E   **True**

(Further details can be found in the *Companion to Psychiatric Studies*, pp. 454–455.)

16.8 **Studies of functional brain imaging have established links between:**

A   Post-traumatic stress disorder and the sensory association cortex.

B   Anorexia nervosa and reduced parietal cortex metabolism.

C   Organic memory impairment and increased hippocampal perfusion.

D   Alzheimer's disease and a regional reduction of blood flow in the parietotemporal cortex.

E   Vascular dementia and focal cortical hypoperfusion.

16.9 **Regarding in vivo binding studies:**

A   Using ^{123}I as a ligand label for single photon emission tomography (SPECT) alters drug (ligand) binding properties.

B   Radioligands are required to have high binding affinity for the receptor site.

C   Regional washout of radioligand is fastest in regions with little non-specific binding.

D   A low signal-to-noise ratio occurs when there is good binding affinity of the radioligand to the specific receptor.

E   High specific binding affinity enables pharmacologically inert amounts of radioligand to be used.

16.10 **In vivo measurement of drug binding at therapeutic doses:**

A   May be examined by displacement of the drug by a radioligand.

B   Has shown that a receptor occupancy of 70–80% is optimal for antipsychotic therapeutic efficacy.

C   Has shown the 5-hydroxytryptamine (5-HT) binding of clozapine to resemble that of haloperidol.

D   Suggests that dopaminergic transmission is increased in depression.

E   Has shown in Gilles de la Tourette syndrome that postsynaptic dopamine receptors are reduced in unmedicated patients.

16.11 **In quantitative scan analysis:**

A   A voxel by voxel method can be used.

B   The region of interest method uses templates to measure average image intensity.

C   Spatial transformation techniques enable images to be compared pixel by pixel.

D   The effect of global activity is a major problem and cannot be removed statistically.

E   Data are filtered to remove variability in gyral anatomy.

(Answers overleaf)

16.8   **A**   **True**   It is probably related to anxious imagery.
            B   **True**   It is possibly associated with cerebral atrophy.
            C   **False**   Perfusion is reduced in the hippocampus in the memory impaired.
            D   **True**   This pattern is thought to be diagnostic.
            E   **True**

(Further details can be found in the *Companion to Psychiatric Studies*, p. 455.)

16.9   **A**   **True**
            B   **True**
            C   **False**   Washout is fastest in regions with much non-specific binding.
            D   **False**   Good binding affinity gives a higher signal.
            E   **True**   < 0.001 mg may be sufficient.

(Further details can be found in the *Companion to Psychiatric Studies*, p. 456.)

16.10   **A**   **True**
            B   **True**   > 80% is associated with side-effects.
            C   **False**   5-HT binding of clozapine is similar to that of risperidone.
            D   **False**   Dopaminergic transmission may be reduced in depression.
            E   **False**   Dopamine reuptake sites may be reduced but postsynaptic receptors are normal.

(Further details can be found in the *Companion to Psychiatric Studies*, pp. 456.)

16.11   **A**   **True**
            B   **True**
            C   **True**
            D   **False**   Global activity can be controlled for statistically.
            E   **True**

(Further details can be found in the *Companion to Psychiatric Studies*, p. 456.)

16.12   Statistical parametric mapping (SPM):

A   Produces a unidimensional representation of brain areas with significant effects.

B   Takes into account the smoothness of the data.

C   Can be used only if a prior hypothesis has been formulated.

D   Can be a fully automated procedure.

E   Can be used in the analysis of structural MRI images.

16.13   Transcranial magnetic stimulation (TMS):

A   Uses a magnetic field to induce electric currents in cortical neurones.

B   Has been in use since the 1960s to measure sensory cortical function.

C   Is able to map cortical function to within a few millimetres.

D   Is capable of demonstrating a causal relationship between local cortical stimulation and functional response.

E   When repeated over frontal areas has been shown to enhance learning.

(Answers overleaf)

16.12 A **False** SPM produces a three-dimensional representation.
      B **True**
      C **False** Differences are displayed where they occur, disregarding any anatomical or preconceived boundary.
      D **True** SPM is fully automated.
      E **True** See, for example, Wright et al 1995.

(Further details can be found in the *Companion to Psychiatric Studies*, p. 457.)

16.13 A **True**
      B **False** TMS has only been in use since the 1980s.
      C **True**
      D **True** This is because it induces the cortical stimulation itself.
      E **False** Repeated TMS (rTMS) over relevant frontal areas disrupts learning.

(Further details can be found in the *Companion to Psychiatric Studies*, p. 461.)

17. Neurotic disorders

17.1   **Regarding neurosis as a general category:**
   A   The term 'neurosis' was coined by Freud.
   B   The term is absent in DSM-IV.
   C   The term is excluded from the ICD-10 classification.
   D   Females outnumber males.
   E   It is less common than psychosis.

17.2   **The National Psychiatric Morbidity Household Survey (NPMS):**
   A   Was conducted in the USA.
   B   Used the Structural Clinical Interview for DSM-IIIR (SCID).
   C   Found fatigue to be the most common neurotic symptom in the population.
   D   Found the total rate of neurotic disorder to be 30%.
   E   Found obsessive–compulsive disorder (OCD) to be the commonest neurotic disorder.

17.3   **Good outcome factors in community samples of patients with neurosis include:**
   A   Physical illness.
   B   Being older.
   C   Severe symptoms at onset.
   D   Being male.
   E   Stable social support.

17.4   **Risk factors identified by Brown for depressive illness in women include:**
   A   Five or more children under the age of 14 years old at home.
   B   Loss of mother before the age of 14 years.
   C   Unemployment.
   D   Low dietary vitamin intake.
   E   Overclose relationship with partner.

(Answers overleaf)   **137**

17.1   A   **False**   It was introduced in 1769 by Cullen, an Edinburgh physician.
       B   **True**
       C   **False**   It was excluded from DSM-IV; it remains in ICD-10.
       D   **True**   The ratio is 2 : 1.
       E   **False**   It is massively more common; prevalence 5–20% of population.

(Further details can be found in the *Companion to Psychiatric Studies*, pp. 465–466.)

17.2   A   **False**   It was conducted in the UK.
       B   **False**   It used the Clinical Interview Schedule (CIS).
       C   **True**
       D   **False**   The rate was 16%.
       E   **False**   OCD was least common with a prevalence of about 1%.

(Further details can be found in the *Companion to Psychiatric Studies*, pp. 470.)

17.3   A   **False**   Physical illness was associated with poorer outcome.
       B   **False**
       C   **False**
       D   **True**
       E   **True**

(Further details can be found in the *Companion to Psychiatric Studies*, p. 472.)

17.4   A   **False**   Three or more children under the age of 14 was the factor identified by Brown.
       B   **True**
       C   **True**
       D   **False**   All of Brown's factors are social factors.
       E   **False**

(Further details can be found in the *Companion to Psychiatric Studies*, p. 472.)

17.5   **The arousal response includes:**
   A   Increased heart rate.
   B   Increased finger pulse volume.
   C   Increased electromyogram (EMG) response.
   D   Increased alpha pattern on an electroencephalogram (EEG).
   E   Increased habituation of the galvanic skin response (GSR).

17.6   **Regarding childhood and neurotic illness:**
   A   More girls have neurosis than boys.
   B   Most childhood illness persists into adulthood.
   C   Thumb-sucking is associated with childhood neurosis.
   D   Childhood schizoid traits usually persist into adulthood.
   E   Unusually close father–son relationship in childhood is linked to adult neurosis.

17.7   **Generalised anxiety disorder (GAD) is associated with:**
   A   Worry of specific content.
   B   Being less fatiguable with exertion.
   C   A later age of onset than in panic disorder.
   D   DSM-IV diagnosis requiring persistent symptoms for 2 weeks.
   E   Attendance at medical clinics.

17.8   **The following are useful in the differential diagnosis of anxiety disorders:**
   A   Lid lag.
   B   Calcium and phosphate.
   C   Glucose.
   D   The level of metadrenalin in the cerebrospinal fluid.
   E   Electrocardiography.

(Answers overleaf)

17.5 A True
     B False   Finger pulse volume is reduced.
     C True
     D False   An EEG shows reduced alpha and increased beta
                pattern.
     E False   There is reduced habituation on GSR.

(Further details can be found in the *Companion to Psychiatric Studies*, p. 475.)

17.6 A False   The sex distribution in children is the reverse of that
                in adults – more boys than girls have neurosis.
     B False   Prospective studies find little continuity.
     C False
     D True
     E False   An unusually close father–son relationship is
                associated with non-neurotic high achievers.

(Further details can be found in the *Companion to Psychiatric Studies*, p. 475.)

17.7 A False   The uncontrollable nature of the worry is specific.
     B False   GAD is associated with being more easily fatigued.
     C False   The age of onset is earlier than in panic disorder.
     D False   DSM-IV requires symptoms of at least 4 weeks'
                duration.
     E True   Patients attend with somatic symptoms.

(Further details can be found in the *Companion to Psychiatric Studies*, pp. 479–480.)

17.8 A True   Lid lag is a clinical sign of thyrotoxicosis.
     B True   Calcium and phosphate are abnormal in parathyroid
                disease.
     C True   Urine metadrenalin and glucose are elevated in
                phaeochromocytoma.
     D False
     E True   ECG may detect paroxysmal atrial tachycardia.

(Further details can be found in the *Companion to Psychiatric Studies*, p. 482.)

17.9   Social phobia:

A   Is commoner in females than in males.
B   Rarely has onset before age 20.
C   Is associated with alcohol abuse.
D   Is rarely associated with depression.
E   Is characterised by a belief that others are persecutory.

17.10   In obsessive–compulsive disorder:

A   Females outnumber males.
B   Prevalence is 5–10%.
C   The precipitant is identified in 30%.
D   More than 50% exhibit obsessional slowness.
E   Delayed presentation is rare.

17.11   Somatisation disorder is associated with:

A   Multiple somatic medically unexplained symptoms over a period of not more than 3 months.
B   Conversion symptoms.
C   Alcoholism in first-degree relatives.
D   Anxious preoccupation regarding the possibility of underlying disease.
E   Positive family history in less than 5% of first-degree relatives.

17.12   In conversion disorder:

A   There may be anaesthesia.
B   La belle indifference is a key diagnostic feature.
C   There is typically an insidious onset.
D   At follow-up more than half will have developed organic disease.
E   The patient has anxious preoccupation about underlying disease.

17.13   The following are typical features of post-traumatic stress disorder:

A   Delayed onset.
B   Anticipatory anxiety.
C   Hypervigilance.
D   Hypersomnia.
E   Incongruous affect.

(Answers overleaf)

17.9   A   **False**   The sex incidence is equal.
      B   **False**   It rarely begins after age 30.
      C   **True**   There is an association with alcohol abuse.
      D   **False**   There is a strong association with depression.
      E   **False**   In the social phobic, realistic fears of ridicule are exaggerated.

(Further details can be found in the *Companion to Psychiatric Studies*, pp. 484–485.)

17.10   A   **True**   The female : male ratio is 1.2–2.3 : 1.
      B   **False**   Prevalence is 2–3%.
      C   **False**   No precipitant is identified in 30%.
      D   **False**   Only 3–4% exhibit obsessional slowness.
      E   **False**   Delayed presentation is typical.

(Further details can be found in the *Companion to Psychiatric Studies*, p. 490.)

17.11   A   **False**   Symptoms are present for much longer.
      B   **True**   They are associated but not essential for diagnosis.
      C   **True**   The family history is of both alcoholism and psychopathy.
      D   **False**   This is hypochondriasis.
      E   **False**   There is a family history of a similar condition in 20%.

(Further details can be found in the *Companion to Psychiatric Studies*, pp. 494–495.)

17.12   A   **True**   The range of symptoms characterised by alteration of sensory or motor function.
      B   **False**   It is not consistently present.
      C   **False**   Onset is typically sudden in relation to a stress.
      D   **False**   Early studies suggested this but not more recent ones.
      E   **False**   This is more typical of hypochondriasis.

(Further details can be found in the *Companion to Psychiatric Studies*, pp. 495–497.)

17.13   A   **True**
      B   **False**   Anticipatory anxiety is a feature of phobic disorder.
      C   **True**
      D   **False**   Reduced sleep is common.
      E   **False**   Numbed affect may be present.

(Further details can be found in the *Companion to Psychiatric Studies*, pp. 501–502.)

18. Eating disorders

18.1 **Anorexia nervosa:**
- A   Is a disorder specific to females only.
- B   Occurs most commonly in adolescent girls and young women.
- C   Cannot be diagnosed in children.
- D   Can rarely affect postmenopausal women.
- E   Affects adolescent boys and young men rarely.

18.2 **The following statements regarding anorexia nervosa are correct:**
- A   There is body-image distortion.
- B   There is loss of sexual interest and potency in men.
- C   The presence of self-induced vomiting excludes a diagnosis of anorexia nervosa.
- D   The presence of self-induced purging excludes a diagnosis of anorexia nervosa.
- E   Excessive exercise may be a feature.

18.3 **The following may be found in association with anorexia nervosa:**
- A   Elevated levels of growth hormone
- B   Raised cortisol levels.
- C   Markedly diminished levels of growth hormone.
- D   Abnormalities of insulin secretion.
- E   Changes in the peripheral metabolism of thyroid hormone.

18.4 **The following are recognised cardiovascular consequences of anorexia nervosa:**
- A   Bradycardia.
- B   Hypertension.
- C   Sudden death.
- D   Mitral valve dysfunction.
- E   Aortic stenosis.

18.5 **The following are recognised consequences of bulimia nervosa:**
- A   Generalised seizures.
- B   Osteoporosis.
- C   Pancreatitis.
- D   Viral hepatitis.
- E   Renal calculi.

(Answers overleaf)   **143**

18.1 A **False** Anorexia nervosa affects both sexes although it is commoner in females.
      B **True**
      C **False** It may affect children approaching puberty.
      D **False** It may affect older women up to the menopause.
      E **True**

(Further details can be found in the *Companion to Psychiatric Studies*, pp. 513–518.)

18.2 A **True**
      B **True**
      C **False**
      D **False**
      E **True**

(Further details can be found in the *Companion to Psychiatric Studies*, p. 512.)

18.3 A **True**
      B **True**
      C **False** Levels are elevated.
      D **True**
      E **True**

(Further details can be found in the *Companion to Psychiatric Studies*, p. 512.)

18.4 A **True**   It is a consequence of starvation.
      B **False**
      C **True**   It is a consequence of starvation.
      D **True**   It is a consequence of starvation.
      E **False**

(Further details can be found in the *Companion to Psychiatric Studies*, p. 517.)

18.5 A **True**
      B **True**
      C **True**
      D **False** Nutritional hepatitis may occur as a result of starvation.
      E **True**

(Further details can be found in the *Companion to Psychiatric Studies*, p. 516.)

18.6   The following are recognised haematological complications of anorexia nervosa:

A   Anaemia.
B   Leukocytosis.
C   Thrombocytopenia.
D   Reduced serum complement levels.
E   Bone marrow hyperplasia.

18.7   Characteristic extreme concerns about shape and weight routinely occur in:

A   Anorexia nervosa (restricting subtype).
B   Anorexia nervosa (bulimic subtype).
C   Bulimia nervosa.
D   Binge-eating disorder.
E   Obesity.

18.8   Bulimic episodes are a consistent feature of:

A   Bulimia nervosa.
B   Anorexia nervosa (restricting subtype).
C   Anorexia nervosa (bulimic subtype).
D   Binge-eating disorder.
E   Obesity.

18.9   Low weight in relation to population norms is always a feature of:

A   Bulimia nervosa.
B   Binge-eating disorder.
C   Anorexia nervosa (restricting subtype).
D   Anorexia nervosa (bulimic subtype).
F   Atypical bulimia nervosa.

18.10   The following are required for a definite diagnosis of bulimia nervosa:

A   A persistent preoccupation with eating and an irresistible craving for food.
B   A morbid dread of fatness.
C   Episodes of overeating in the form of a binge.
D   Body weight maintained at a level below that expected from population norms.
E   Amenorrhoea.

(Answers overleaf)

18.6   A   True
        B   False
        C   True
        D   True
        E   False

(Further details can be found in the *Companion to Psychiatric Studies*, p. 516.)

18.7   A   True
        B   True
        C   True
        D   False
        E   False

(Further details can be found in the *Companion to Psychiatric Studies*, p. 511.)

18.8   A   True
        B   False
        C   True
        D   True
        E   False

(Further details can be found in the *Companion to Psychiatric Studies*, p. 511.)

18.9   A   False
        B   False
        C   True
        D   True
        E   False

(Further details can be found in the *Companion to Psychiatric Studies*, p. 511.)

18.10   A   True
        B   True
        C   True
        D   False   Body weight may range from being underweight to overweight.
        E   False   This is a feature of anorexia nervosa.

(Further details can be found in the *Companion to Psychiatric Studies*, pp. 511 and 521.)

18.11   Repeated vomiting associated with bulimia nervosa may result in:
A   Tetany.
B   Dental erosions.
C   Epileptic seizures.
D   Cardiac arrhythmias.
E   Muscular weakness.

18.12   Starvation may lead to the following metabolic complications:
A   Impaired temperature regulation.
B   Hypercholesterolaemia.
C   Hypocarotenaemia.
D   Impaired glucose tolerance.
E   Hypoproteinaemia.

18.13   The following have a specific role in the aetiology of bulimia nervosa:
A   Family history of obesity.
B   Personal history of obesity.
C   Family history of substance abuse.
D   Family history of affective disorders.
E   Childhood sexual abuse.

18.14   The following are recognised physical complications of bulimia nervosa:
A   Oesophageal perforation.
B   Mallory–Weiss tears.
C   Gastric shrinkage.
D   Acne.
E   Electrolyte abnormalities.

(Answers overleaf)

18.11   A   True
         B   True
         C   True
         D   True
         E   True

(Further details can be found in the *Companion to Psychiatric Studies*, p. 524.)

18.12   A   True
         B   True
         C   False
         D   True
         E   True

(Further details can be found in the *Companion to Psychiatric Studies*, p. 516.)

18.13   A   True
         B   True
         C   True
         D   True
         E   False   It is a non-specific risk factor for psychiatric disorder in general.

(Further details can be found in the *Companion to Psychiatric Studies*, p. 525.)

18.14   A   True
         B   True
         C   False   Gastric dilatation is a recognised complication.
         D   False   There is no evidence for this.
         E   True

(Further details can be found in the *Companion to Psychiatric Studies*, p. 524.)

19. Sexual disorders

19.1 **Erectile dysfunction:**
  A Has a clear relationship with age.
  B Is the second commonest reason for men to present to a sexual problems service.
  C Affects 50% of men aged over 40 years.
  D Is unrelated to general health status.
  E Is a recognised result of venous incompetence.

19.2 **Sexual dysfunction:**
  A Is equally common in male and female diabetic patients.
  B Affects one-third of male medical outpatients.
  C Is more likely in patients with hypertension.
  D Is more likely in patients on renal dialysis.
  E May be caused by the effect of anticonvulsant medication on plasma free testosterone.

19.3 **Penile erection depends on:**
  A Contraction of the smooth muscle in the corpora cavernosa.
  B Increase of venous outflow.
  C Increase in arterial inflow.
  D A build-up of pressure close to diastolic pressure within the corpora.
  E Sufficient arterial supply from the pelvic arteries.

19.4 **Sex therapy:**
  A Is effective for vaginismus.
  B Patients with orgasmic dysfunction have the worst outcome.
  C Includes sensate focus therapy.
  D Includes didactic teaching about anatomy and physiology.
  E Involves setting 'homework' for patients.

(Answers overleaf)

19.1 A **True**   It is more than twice as prevalent in the over-50s as in the under-50s.

   B **False**   It is the presenting problem for more than two-thirds of presentations.

   C **True**   Only 48% of men over 40 years old denied any problems with erections.

   D **False**   Most reported sexual difficulties have a relationship with general health.

   E **True**   The erectile tissue fails to occlude venous drainage during the development of an erection.

(Further details can be found in the *Companion to Psychiatric Studies*, pp. 529 and 532.)

19.2 A **False**   It affects up to 50% of male diabetics but very few female diabetics.

   B **True**
   C **True**
   D **True**
   E **True**   Anticonvulsant medication may reduce testosterone, resulting in lowered sexual interest.

(Further details can be found in the *Companion to Psychiatric Studies*, pp. 531–532.)

19.3 A **False**   It depends on relaxation of the smooth muscle in the corpora cavernosa.

   B **False**   It depends on reduction of venous outflow.
   C **True**
   D **False**   The pressure build-up is close to systolic pressure.
   E **True**

(Further details can be found in the *Companion to Psychiatric Studies*, p. 532.)

19.4 A **True**
   B **False**   Low desire has worst outcome.
   C **True**
   D **True**
   E **True**

(Further details can be found in the *Companion to Psychiatric Studies*, pp. 536–537.)

19.5   The following drug treatments work by direct local effects:

A   Papaverine.
B   Yohimbine.
C   Prostaglandin E.
D   Alprostadil.
E   Sildenafil.

19.6   The following statements regarding the development of sexual orientation are correct:

A   Homosexual behaviour is commonplace amongst non-human primates.
B   Exclusive homosexual preference is confined to humans.
C   Twin studies do not support genetic factors as being important in homosexuality.
D   There is recent evidence of a link between a Y chromosome marker and homosexual orientation in men.
E   Hormonal factors are highly likely to be involved in the development of sexual orientation in men.

19.7   The following statements about genital responses are correct:

A   They rely predominantly on vasocongestion in men.
B   They do not rely predominantly on vasocongestion in women.
C   The pathophysiology of erection at the level of the penis remains unclear.
D   The majority of postmenopausal women experience vaginal dryness secondary to oestrogen deficiency.
E   Dyspareunia in women is commonly caused by vaginal infections or deep pelvic pathology.

19.8   The following statements concerning exhibitionism are correct:

A   Exhibitionists are often referred for psychiatric help.
B   In exhibitionism the victim's response is unimportant.
C   Indecent exposure associated with learning disability is often aimed at establishing further sexual contact.
D   Exhibitionist behaviour is more likely to persist if associated with sexual arousal at the thought of exposure than if not.
E   Marital sexual problems are common amongst exhibitionists.

(Answers overleaf)

19.5 A **True** It is a smooth muscle relaxant injected into the corpora cavernosa of the penis.

B **False** Yohimbine has a centrally acting action.

C **True** Prostaglandin E_1 can be given by intracavernosal injection or intraurethral application.

D **True**

E **False** Sildenafil acts by phosphodiesterase inhibition.

(Further details can be found in the *Companion to Psychiatric Studies*, p. 539.)

19.6 A **True**

B **True**

C **False** Twin pair and family pedigree studies strongly suggest a genetic factor.

D **False** Evidence is linked to an X chromosome marker.

E **False**

(Further details can be found in the *Companion to Psychiatric Studies*, p. 541.)

19.7 A **True**

B **False** Genital responses rely predominantly on vasocongestion in both men and women.

C **False** This has been extensively researched.

D **False** The majority of postmenopausal women appear to have enough oestrogen to avoid this problem.

E **True**

(Further details can be found in the *Companion to Psychiatric Studies*, p. 532.)

19.8 A **True**

B **False** The reaction of the victim is important and an exhibitionist may go on exposing until he produces the desired response.

C **True**

D **True**

E **True**

(Further details can be found in the *Companion to Psychiatric Studies*, p. 545.)

19.9   **With regard to sexual offenders:**

A   Cognitive behaviour therapy (CBT) has been shown to be the most effective treatment in repeat offenders.

B   The legal process is generally ineffective.

C   A minority of sexual offenders are deterred by their first conviction.

D   Oestrogens are the drugs of first choice in the pharmacological treatment of sexual offenders.

E   Drugs are mainly used to induce erectile failure.

19.10   **Physical investigations of sexual dysfunction are particularly indicated if the patient presents with:**

A   Recent loss of sexual interest in the absence of a psychological explanation.

B   Pain.

C   Erectile dysfunction with morning erections still present.

D   An acute sexual problem.

E   Premature ejaculation.

19.11   **The following statements regarding physical treatments for transsexualism are correct:**

A   Oestrogens enhance sexual interest and response.

B   Oestrogens slow body hair growth.

C   Androgen therapy can result in clitoral atrophy.

D   Urinary fistulae are a particular problem for male to female transsexuals.

E   The vaginal barrel is more often fashioned from skin than from colon.

(Answers overleaf)

19.9 A **False** CBT is most effective in first-time offenders.

B **False** The large majority of sexual offenders are deterred by their first conviction.

C **False**

D **False** The use of oestrogens has been superseded by the antiandrogen, cyproterone acetate.

E **False** These drugs are used to reduce sexual interest.

(Further details can be found in the *Companion to Psychiatric Studies*, p. 546.)

19.10 A **True**

B **True**

C **False** The continuation of erections on waking in this setting is a useful indicator of psychogenic causation.

D **False**

E **False**

(Further details can be found in the *Companion to Psychiatric Studies*, p. 535.)

19.11 A **False** Oestrogens may suppress sexual interest and response.

B **True**

C **False** Clitoral enlargement is to be expected with androgen therapy.

D **False** The surgical creation of a penis can be associated with urinary fistulae.

E **True**

(Further details can be found in the *Companion to Psychiatric Studies*, p. 547.)

20. Women's disorders

20.1 **The premenstrual syndrome (PMS):**
- **A** Is associated with symptoms occurring between ovulation and the onset of menstruation.
- **B** May present with symptoms during any phase of the menstrual cycle.
- **C** Is a cyclical disorder in girls occurring prior to the menstrual cycle being established.
- **D** Has only a weak association with depressive disorder.
- **E** Occurs in less than 2% of women.

20.2 **Evidence-based treatments for premenstrual syndrome include:**
- **A** Progesterone.
- **B** Magnesium.
- **C** Vitamin C.
- **D** Danazol.
- **E** Antidepressants.

20.3 **Regarding postmenopausal disorders:**
- **A** Postmenopausal women are at greater risk of developing depressive disorders.
- **B** It has been proposed that prolonged perimenopausal exposure to oestrogen can exacerbate mood disturbance.
- **C** Postmenopausal depression has been proven to be due to the stress of ageing.
- **D** Oestrogen replacement is the treatment of choice for all affected women.
- **E** Perimenopausal depression is best treated with antidepressant drugs.

(Answers overleaf)

20.1   A   **True**
      B   **False**   Symptoms occur between ovulation and menstruation.
      C   **False**   It is a menstrual disorder.
      D   **False**   30–40% of women with PMS have depressive disorders.
      E   **False**   40% meet recognised criteria and 3–8% meet criteria which include impaired functioning.

(Further details can be found in the *Companion to Psychiatric Studies*, pp. 552–553.)

20.2   A   **False**   It was no more effective than placebo in randomised trials.
      B   **True**   There is some randomised controlled trial (RCT) evidence.
      C   **False**   There is no good evidence.
      D   **True**   It suppresses ovulation.
      E   **True**   There is good RCT evidence.

(Further details can be found in the *Companion to Psychiatric Studies*, p. 554.)

20.3   A   **False**   It is a commonly held view but is not supported by evidence.
      B   **True**   There is some evidence for this.
      C   **False**   The association has been proposed but is unproven.
      D   **False**   The effect on mood disorder is not proven.
      E   **True**

(Further details can be found in the *Companion to Psychiatric Studies*, p. 556.)

20.4   Normal pregnancy is associated with:
A   A significant increase in rates of mental disorder in teenagers.
B   Anxiety and depression in the second trimester.
C   Increased anxiety and depression in the first and third trimester.
D   An increased rate of psychiatric disorders.
E   Onset of schizophrenia.

20.5   In depression associated with pregnancy:
A   Treatment should focus on psychosocial intervention in the first instance.
B   Electroconvulsive therapy (ECT) is contraindicated.
C   Progesterone is helpful.
D   Secondary amine tricyclics (e.g. nortriptyline) are contraindicated.
E   Anticonvulsant mood stabilisers are useful preventive agents

20.6   Therapeutic abortions are associated with:
A   No increased rates of psychiatric morbidity.
B   A grief reaction or depressive disorder in more than 50% of women.
C   A high rate of chronic psychiatric morbidity.
D   A greater risk of disorder where abortion conflicts with religious beliefs.
E   Onset of obsessive–compulsive disorder (OCD).

20.7   Hyperemesis gravidarum:
A   Affects about 10% of pregnant women.
B   Is a condition associated with severe diarrhoea.
C   Has a peak incidence at 8–12 weeks of pregnancy.
D   Is less common in women with a history of gastroenterological disorder.
E   Is a condition in which antiemetics are contraindicated.

(Answers overleaf)

20.4   **A**   **True**   However, there is no significant increase in rates of mental disorder in older women.

          B   **False**   The first and third trimesters show some increase, not the second.

          C   **True**

          D   **False**   The rate is increased only in teenagers and those with pre-existing disorders.

          E   **False**   There is no evidence for this.

(Further details can be found in the *Companion to Psychiatric Studies*, p. 556.)

20.5   **A**   **True**   For example, appropriate treatments are those that enhance adjustment or provide support.

          B   **False**   ECT is indicated for severe depression.

          C   **False**

          D   **False**   They are considered relatively safe.

          E   **False**   They are associated with fetal abnormality.

(Further details can be found in the *Companion to Psychiatric Studies*, pp. 556 and 561.)

20.6   **A**   **False**   There is an increase – especially in the first month after the event.

          B   **True**

          C   **False**   It is usually transient.

          D   **True**

          E   **False**   There is no evidence for this.

(Further details can be found in the *Companion to Psychiatric Studies*, p. 556.)

20.7   **A**   **False**   It affects only about 1% of pregnant women.

          B   **False**   It is associated with nausea and vomiting.

          C   **True**

          D   **False**   It is more common in women with a history of gastroenterological disorder.

          E   **False**   They should be used cautiously.

(Further details can be found in the *Companion to Psychiatric Studies*, pp. 556–557.)

20.8   **Maternity blues:**
  A   Has an onset 10–30 days after childbirth.
  B   Affects between 30 and 80% of women following childbirth.
  C   Is associated with complications at delivery.
  D   Is associated with depression in the last trimester of pregnancy.
  E   Is best treated with oestrogen injections.

20.9   **The prescription of antidepressant drugs is often necessary in the following disorders:**
  A   Maternity blues.
  B   Postnatal depression.
  C   Postpartum psychosis.
  D   Hyperemesis gravidarum.
  E   Pseudocyesis.

20.10   **Postnatal depression:**
  A   Affects 10–15% of women following childbirth.
  B   Is a transient, self-limiting disorder.
  C   Typically occurs in the first week following childbirth.
  D   Differs in nature and course from other types of depressive disorder.
  E   Is another term for maternity blues.

20.11   **The following increase the risk of postnatal depression:**
  A   A complicated obstetric history.
  B   Severe maternity blues.
  C   High social class.
  D   Family history of affective disorder.
  E   Personal history of thyroid disease.

20.12   **Postpartum psychosis:**
  A   Has a rapid onset within 48 hours after childbirth.
  B   Usually has a very gradual onset.
  C   Is associated with increased risk of hospitalisation for psychosis for 2 years.
  D   Has a second incidence peak 1–3 months following delivery.
  E   Affects 5% of women following childbirth.

(Answers overleaf)

20.8   A   **False**   Its onset is 3–10 days after childbirth.
        B   **True**
        C   **False**
        D   **True**
        E   **False**   A hormonal aetiology is unproven and there is no good evidence that this helpful.

(Further details can be found in the *Companion to Psychiatric Studies*, p. 557.)

20.9   A   **False**   Maternity blues is a transient, self-limiting disorder.
        B   **True**   Severe cases may require electroconvulsive therapy.
        C   **True**   There are often affective features; it may also require antipsychotic drugs.
        D   **False**   Treatment is mainly symptomatic.
        E   **False**   Treatment is usually psychological.

(Further details can be found in the *Companion to Psychiatric Studies*, pp. 556–559.)

20.10   A   **True**
        B   **False**
        C   **False**   It develops insidiously 3–4 weeks after childbirth.
        D   **False**
        E   **False**   Blues is a mild early transient condition.

(Further details can be found in the *Companion to Psychiatric Studies*, pp. 557–558.)

20.11   A   **False**
        B   **True**
        C   **False**
        D   **True**
        E   **False**

(Further details can be found in the *Companion to Psychiatric Studies*, p. 558.)

20.12   A   **False**   Onset is rarely so early, but is usually in the first 1–2 weeks.
        B   **False**   Onset is usually rapid.
        C   **True**
        D   **True**
        E   **False**   It is a rare but serious disorder affecting 0.2% of women following childbirth.

(Further details can be found in the *Companion to Psychiatric Studies*, pp. 560–561.)

20.13   The following statements are true regarding the presentation of postpartum psychosis:

A   Worsening insomnia is a common prodromal symptom.

B   80% of those affected present with paranoid syndromes.

C   The most common presentation is schizophreniform.

D   In those that present with affective symptoms, depressive symptoms predominate.

E   Infanticide is common.

(Answers overleaf)

20.13 **A** **True**
       B **False** 80% present with affective symptoms.
       C **False** The most common presentation is with affective symptoms – 80%.
       D **False** Half of the affective cases present with features of mania.
       E **False** Infanticide is a rare association.

(Further details can be found in the *Companion to Psychiatric Studies*, p. 560.)

21. Personality

21.1 Considering approaches to 'normal' personality:
- A Freudian personality theory may be considered as nomothetic.
- B Self-actualisation theory is a humanistic approach to personality theory.
- C Trait theory takes Maslow's hierarchy of needs into account.
- D Astrology encompasses a type-based personality classification.
- E Eysenck's personality traits are an example of a nomothetic approach.

21.2 The following are associated with trait personality theory:
- A Eysenck.
- B Cattel.
- C Costa and McCrae.
- D Cloninger.
- E Rogers.

21.3 Trait personality theory:
- A Includes cognitive–behavioural models.
- B Is associated with measurement of personality using the Eysenck Personality Questionnaire.
- C Predicts continuity of behavioural response over time.
- D Has limited research evidence in its favour.
- E Led to the development of Rogerian client-centred therapy.

21.4 In Eysenck's three factor theory of personality:
- A The dimensions measured are narrow.
- B Extraversion shows a low heritability.
- C Psychoticism includes impulsivity.
- D The dimensions are thought to be related to distinct biological factors.
- E The dimension of neuroticism follows a normal distribution in the general population.

(Answers overleaf)

21.1   A   **False**   Freudian theory is idiographic.
      B   **True**   It focuses on human growth and potential.
      C   **False**   Maslow's theories are idiographic.
      D   **True**
      E   **True**

(Further details can be found in the *Companion to Psychiatric Studies*, pp. 565–567.)

21.2   A   **True**   Eysenck is associated with the three factor theory.
      B   **True**   Cattel is associated with the sixteen factor theory.
      C   **True**   Costa and McCrae proposed the five factor model.
      D   **True**   Cloninger proposed the seven factor model.
      E   **False**   Rogers is associated with self-actualisation.

(Further details can be found in the *Companion to Psychiatric Studies*, pp. 567–570.)

21.3   A   **False**   This is idiographic.
      B   **True**
      C   **True**
      D   **False**
      E   **False**   Rogerian therapy is humanistic, i.e. idiographic.

(Further details can be found in the *Companion to Psychiatric Studies*, pp. 568–569.)

21.4   A   **False**   They are very broad.
      B   **False**   It has a moderately high heritability.
      C   **True**
      D   **True**   Extraversion is thought to be linked to arousal, neuroticism to reactivity.
      E   **True**

(Further details can be found in the *Companion to Psychiatric Studies*, pp. 569–570.)

21.5   Situationalist theory of personality:
A   Is largely associated with the work of Mischel.
B   Is supported by the poor correlation between personality trait and behaviour.
C   Takes behavioural aggregation into account.
D   Predicts cross-situational consistency.
E   Is incompatible with trait theory.

21.6   Regarding genetic factors in personality:
A   Studies show inherited factors are more important than family environment.
B   Extraversion traits are at least 50% due to inherited factors.
C   Individual experiences are more important in determining personality.
D   Monozygotic twin personality trait correlation has been found to be more than twice that of dizygotic twin trait correlation.
E   Variations in the 5-HT transporter gene have been shown to be associated with neuroticism traits.

21.7   Personality disorder:
A   Shows continuity between normal personality theory and disorder classification.
B   Probably results more from early experiences than genetic factors.
C   Follows a nomothetic classification.
D   Should not be diagnosed in the presence of a major psychiatric disorder.
E   Classification arises mainly from behavioural psychology.

21.8   The following are true of schizoid personality disorder:
A   The concept includes restricted affective expression.
B   Twin studies suggest a link with schizophrenia.
C   Patients are characterised by impoverished social relationships.
D   When using DSM-IV criteria, it has a prevalence of ~ 15% amongst psychiatric outpatients.
E   The presentation has a large overlap with avoidant personality disorder.

(Answers overleaf)

21.5 A **True**
  B **True** Personality traits rarely correlate with behaviours above 0.3.
  C **False** Behavioural aggregations over several situations suggests dispositions.
  D **False**
  E **False** A compromise of interaction between traits and situations is now accepted.

(Further details can be found in the *Companion to Psychiatric Studies*, pp. 573–574.)

21.6 A **True**
  B **False** The heritability of extraversion is about 32–36%.
  C **False** Genetic factors are the most important.
  D **True**
  E **False**

(Further details can be found in the *Companion to Psychiatric Studies*, pp. 574–576.)

21.7 A **False** Disorders are categories.
  B **False**
  C **True**
  D **False** See, for example, Axes I and II of DSM-IV.
  E **False** It arises from clinical observation.

(Further details can be found in the *Companion to Psychiatric Studies*, pp. 576–578.)

21.8 A **True**
  B **False**
  C **True**
  D **True**
  E **True**

(Further details can be found in the *Companion to Psychiatric Studies*, pp. 578–579.)

21.9 **The following personality disorders and diagnoses are associated correctly:**

A   Avoidant personality disorder – social phobia.
B   Schizoid personality disorder – schizophrenia.
C   Narcissistic personality disorder – mania.
D   Borderline personality disorder – alcohol abuse.
E   Histrionic personality disorder – agoraphobia.

21.10 **The following features support a diagnosis of schizotypal personality disorder:**

A   Previous episodes of depressive illness.
B   A pattern of social avoidance.
C   Schneiderian first rank symptoms.
D   Presence of ideas of reference.
E   Negative features of schizophrenia.

21.11 **The following are characteristic of antisocial personality disorder:**

A   Addiction.
B   Criminality.
C   Underlying low self-esteem.
D   Impulsivity.
E   Lack of remorse.

21.12 **Borderline personality disorder:**

A   Requires three criteria for impulsive personality disorder to be met in ICD-10.
B   Is part of the fearful/anxious cluster in DSM-IV.
C   Is found in ~ 2% of the general population.
D   Is characterised by disturbance of self-identity.
E   Results in emotionally cold relationships.

21.13 **Avoidant personality disorder:**

A   Is distinguishable from social phobia by time course.
B   Is characterised by avoidance of interpersonal contact.
C   Results from underlying emotional coldness.
D   Is present in ~ 10% of psychiatric outpatients.
E   Is characterised by fear of criticism or rejection.

(Answers overleaf)

21.9   A   True
       B   False
       C   False
       D   False
       E   False

(Further details can be found in the *Companion to Psychiatric Studies*, pp. 578–586.)

21.10 A   True
       B   True
       C   False
       D   True
       E   True

(Further details can be found in the *Companion to Psychiatric Studies*, p. 579.)

21.11 A   False
       B   True
       C   False
       D   True
       E   True

(Further details can be found in the *Companion to Psychiatric Studies*, pp. 579–580.)

21.12 A   True
       B   True
       C   True
       D   True
       E   False   Relationships are typically unstable.

(Further details can be found in the *Companion to Psychiatric Studies*, pp. 580–581.)

21.13 A   False   Social phobia may be continuous (see *Companion to Psychiatric Studies*, p. 586).
       B   True
       C   False   It may result from anxiety or narcissistic vulnerability.
       D   True
       E   True

(Further details can be found in the *Companion to Psychiatric Studies*, p. 583.)

21.14 **With respect to pharmacotherapy in borderline personality disorder:**

A   There is no evidence of efficacy of monoamine oxidase inhibitors (MAOIs).

B   Benzodiazepines are useful in managing acute crises.

C   Selective serotonin reuptake inhibitors (SSRIs) can be useful as a maintenance treatment.

D   Carbamazepine can control mood swings.

E   SSRIs may reduce some undesirable behaviour.

(Answers overleaf)

21.14 **A** **False** There is evidence of efficacy in acute crises.
        B **True**
        C **False** There is no proven effective maintenance treatment.
        D **False** See C above.
        E **True**

(Further details can be found in the *Companion to Psychiatric Studies*, p. 592.)

22. Learning disability

22.1 **The following statements regarding historical aspects of the concept of learning disability are true:**
- **A** English legislation first differentiated mental illness and learning disability during the reign of Edward I.
- **B** Séguin first introduced the term congenital amentia.
- **C** Pinel first advanced the idea of acquired and congenital forms of learning disability.
- **D** Pritchard graded the extent of intellectual impairment from profound to normal.
- **E** Mass sterilisation programmes began in some states of the USA as early as 1907.

22.2 **DSM-IV:**
- **A** Codes mental retardation on Axis I.
- **B** Allows for an overall assessment of adaptive functioning on Axis IV.
- **C** Characterises mental retardation as intellectual impairment of IQ 50 or less.
- **D** Specifies that the onset of mental retardation must be before the age of 18.
- **E** Specifies that impairment of adaptive functioning must be present to make the diagnosis of mental retardation.

22.3 **Regarding the prevalence and epidemiology of learning disability:**
- **A** The IQ distribution of the general population is Gaussian.
- **B** 1–2% of the population have an IQ less than 70.
- **C** In 80% of people with mild learning disability (IQ of 50–70) a cause for their learning disability is identifiable.
- **D** In Scandinavian studies, 5% of people with learning disability and an IQ of 50–70 had fetal alcohol syndrome.
- **E** In 10–20% of all people with learning disability a biological cause is identifiable.

(Answers overleaf)

22.1   **A** **False**   It was during the reign of Edward II.
        B **False**   Séguin advocated treatment; Cullen introduced congenital amentia.
        C **True**
        D **True**
        E **True**

(Further details can be found in the *Companion to Psychiatric Studies*, p. 598.)

22.2   **A** **False**   Mental retardation is coded on Axis II.
        B **False**   Axis V allows for an overall assessment of adaptive functioning.
        C **False**   IQ of 70 or less defines mental impairment.
        D **True**
        E **True**

(Further details can be found in the *Companion to Psychiatric Studies*, pp. 599–600.)

22.3   **A** **False**   The distribution is skewed by those with low and very low IQs.
        B **True**
        C **False**   No cause can be found in over 50% of those with mild learning disability.
        D **True**
        E **True**

(Further details can be found in the *Companion to Psychiatric Studies*, p. 600.)

22.4   **Regarding the genetics of Down's syndrome:**

A   The extra chromosome 21 is usually of paternal origin.
B   Most paternal chromosome errors occur in the first meiotic division.
C   Mitotic errors account for 40% of cases.
D   95% of cases have a full trisomy 21.
E   45% of Robertsonian translocations are due to a fusion chromosome.

22.5   **In Down's syndrome:**

A   Cardiac arrhythmia is the commonest cause of death.
B   There is a reduction in the anteroposterior diameter of the head.
C   Instability of the atlanto-axial joint occurs.
D   The immune system is commonly compromised.
E   Diabetes mellitus is commoner than in the normal population.

22.6   **Dementia in Down's syndrome:**

A   Is more common in people with the APOE4 allele.
B   May be reliably diagnosed by a single MRI scan.
C   Renders the individual more susceptible to the development of hyperthyroidism.
D   Is best treated by expedient hospitalisation.
E   Rarely occurs before the age of 50.

22.7   **Klinefelter's syndrome:**

A   Occurs in 1 in 100 000 males.
B   When non-disjunction is paternally derived is associated with paternal age.
C   Is associated with infertility.
D   Is commonly associated with obsessive–compulsive psychopathology.
E   Is usually associated with a moderate degree of learning disability.

(Answers overleaf)

22.4 **A** **False** The extra chromosome is maternal in over 90% of cases.
      B **False** Most maternal errors occur in the first division; paternal errors in the second.
      C **False** Mitotic errors account for about 5% of cases.
      D **True**
      E **True** It is usually between chromosomes 14 and 21.

(Further details can be found in the *Companion to Psychiatric Studies*, pp. 603–604.)

22.5 **A** **False** Infection is the leading cause of death.
      B **True** This is known as brachycephaly.
      C **True** In 1.5% it is due to weakness of the transverse ligament.
      D **True** Antibody levels tend to be raised and T lymphocytes reduced.
      E **True** There may be an autoimmune basis.

(Further details can be found in the *Companion to Psychiatric Studies*, pp. 605–606.)

22.6 **A** **False** This is true of the general population but studies in Down's are conflicting.
      B **False** The diagnosis is clinical.
      C **False** Hypothyroidism may be increased, however.
      D **False** Noise and changing staff probably only increase fear and disorientation.
      E **False** The prevalence is 40% for those over 40.

(Further details can be found in the *Companion to Psychiatric Studies*, pp. 608–610.)

22.7 **A** **False** The prevalence is 1 in 1000 men.
      B **True** It is also true of maternally derived cases.
      C **True**
      D **False** However, there may be a link with psychosis.
      E **False** The average IQ is 90 and most are above 60.

(Further details can be found in the *Companion to Psychiatric Studies*, p. 612.)

22.8   **An autosomal recessive pattern of inheritance occurs in:**
   A   Hunter's disease.
   B   Sialidosis.
   C   Sanfillipo disease.
   D   Fabry's disease.
   E   Niemann–Pick disease.

22.9   **Tuberose sclerosis:**
   A   Affects more males than females.
   B   Has an estimated prevalence of 1 in 10 000.
   C   Is dermatologically characterised by 'beech branch' patches.
   D   Often first presents with 'salaam attacks' in infancy.
   E   Has at least four distinct genotypic forms.

22.10   **Fragile X syndrome:**
   A   Is the commonest inherited disorder associated with learning disability.
   B   Is associated with mitral valve prolapse.
   C   Is associated with micro-orchidism.
   D   Is associated with abnormally small bilateral hippocampi.
   E   May be detected prenatally.

22.11   **Autism:**
   A   Was first described by Leo Kanner.
   B   Has been associated with the 'drinks cabinet' mother.
   C   Cannot be diagnosed if learning disability is present.
   D   Is referred to as a pervasive developmental disorder in ICD-10.
   E   Is defined as having an onset before the age of 5 in ICD-10.

(Answers overleaf)

22.8 A **False** Hunter's disease is an X-linked recessive lysosomal storage disease.
  B **True** Sialidosis is a lysosomal storage disease.
  C **True** Sanfillipo disease is a lysosomal storage disease.
  D **False** Fabry's disease is another X-linked recessive lysosomal storage disease.
  E **True** Niemann–Pick disease is a lysosomal storage disease.

(Further details can be found in the *Companion to Psychiatric Studies*, p. 614.)

22.9 A **False** It is autosomal dominant.
  B **True**
  C **False** Depigmented 'ash leaf spots' are characteristic.
  D **True** These are infantile spasms.
  E **False** Three forms exist – from genes on chromosomes 9, 12 and 16.

(Further details can be found in the *Companion to Psychiatric Studies*, p. 614.)

22.10 A **True** It affects approximately 1 in 4000 males.
  B **True** This is possibly due to a connective tissue disorder.
  C **False** Enlarged testicles – up to 120 ml – are found in 80% of male cases.
  D **False** Affected individuals tend to have slightly enlarged skulls, ventricles, hippocampi and caudate nuclei.
  E **True**

(Further details can be found in the *Companion to Psychiatric Studies*, pp. 615–619.)

22.11 A **True** It was described by Kanner in 1943.
  B **False** The association is with the 'refrigerator mother'.
  C **False** Both diagnoses are made in such cases.
  D **True**
  E **False** Onset before 3 years of age is required.

(Further details can be found in the *Companion to Psychiatric Studies*, p. 622.)

22.12 **Autism:**
A Affects males more often than females.
B May be associated with prolonged eye contact.
C Is associated with echolalia.
D Occurs in 10% of the siblings of an affected proband.
E Is associated with specific deficits in 'theory of mind'.

22.13 **Schizophrenia in people with mild learning disability:**
A Occurs 20 times more often than in the normal population.
B Is characterised by marked thought disorder.
C Is associated with a later age of onset.
D Is associated with a high degree of familiality.
E May be associated with chromosomal rearrangements.

22.14 **Challenging behaviours:**
A Are commonest in people with severe learning disability.
B Are found in 40% of all people with learning disability.
C Are commonest in hospital populations.
D Are commonly associated with mental illness in people with mild learning disability.
E Tend to be short-lived in people with severe learning disability and autistic features.

(Answers overleaf)

22.12   **A**   **True**   Males are two to three times more likely to be affected.
       B   **True**   Long periods of staring may be a feature.
       C   **True**
       D   **False**   The rate is about 3% in siblings.
       E   **True**   The theory postulates difficulty in attributing concepts of mental states to the self and non-self.

(Further details can be found in the *Companion to Psychiatric Studies*, pp. 623–625.)

22.13   **A**   **False**   The rate is 3–6% compared to 1% in the general population.
       B   **False**   Thought disorder is less evident than in schizophrenia.
       C   **False**   The age at onset is earlier.
       D   **True**   There is often a high degree of familiality for both schizophrenia and learning disability.
       E   **True**

(Further details can be found in the *Companion to Psychiatric Studies*, p. 628.)

22.14   **A**   **True**
       B   **False**   The rate is 7% overall.
       C   **True**   The rate is 14% in hospital populations.
       D   **True**
       E   **False**   They tend to be persistent in severe learning disability.

(Further details can be found in the *Companion to Psychiatric Studies*, pp. 630–631.)

23. Psychiatric disorders in childhood

23.1   The following are Piagetian stages of cognitive development:
A   Sensorimotor phase.
B   Flexible operational.
C   Formal operational.
D   Premotor.
E   Genital.

23.2   In Piaget's sensorimotor stage:
A   Average age is ~ 18 months.
B   Thinking is dominated by operations.
C   One main developmental task is object permanence.
D   The child is unable to recognise his or her influence on the environment.
E   Conservation of number starts.

23.3   A child in the preoperational phase will:
A   Be between 8 and 12 years old.
B   Ascribe personalities to inanimate objects.
C   Be able to distinguish self from not self.
D   Display an understanding of others' point of view.
E   Understand events occurring by chance or fate.

23.4   The following are true of Piaget's formal operational period:
A   Typical age is in the teenage years.
B   Ability to reason logically becomes apparent.
C   There is difficulty in abstracting general rules from specific situations.
D   This stage must be completed before adulthood is attained.
E   There is the ability to develop and test hypotheses.

(Answers overleaf)   **179**

23.1 A **True** This stage lasts on average from birth to 2 years.
        B **False** There is a concrete operational stage between the ages of 7 and 12 years.
        C **True** This stage is from 12 years and upwards.
        D **False**
        E **False** It is a Freudian stage.

(Further details can be found in the *Companion to Psychiatric Studies*, pp. 651–653.)

23.2 A **True**
        B **False** Thinking is dominated by innate reflexes.
        C **True** Learning an object still exists even though the object is no longer visible.
        D **False** The child learns this now.
        E **False** It is a task of the preoperational phase.

(Further details can be found in the *Companion to Psychiatric Studies*, pp. 651–652.)

23.3 A **False** The child will be between 2 and 7 years old.
        B **True**
        C **True**
        D **False** This develops during the concrete operational phase – 7–12 years.
        E **False** This develops later.

(Further details can be found in the *Companion to Psychiatric Studies*, pp. 652–653.)

23.4 A **True**
        B **False** It occurs in the previous formal operational period.
        C **False**
        D **False** It is not always attained by adults.
        E **True**

(Further details can be found in the *Companion to Psychiatric Studies*, p. 653.)

23.5   **The following are characteristic of normal social development:**
A   Attachment coincides with stranger anxiety.
B   Social smiling is usually present from around 8 weeks.
C   A child of 6 will have strong friendships without regard to gender.
D   At 8 months, a child will tend to become anxious in the absence of its mother.
E   Lasting relationships become apparent from around 8 years.

23.6   **In the classification of childhood psychiatric disorders:**
A   Classification is more widely used than a phenomenological approach.
B   DSM-IV codes developmental disorder on Axis I.
C   ICD-10 codes mental retardation on Axis II.
D   Conduct disorder is included in both ICD-10 and DSM-IV.
E   Mixed disorders may be separated into conduct or emotional disorders.

23.7   **The following are risk factors in the parent for physical abuse:**
A   Low self-esteem.
B   History of abuse as a child.
C   Single parent.
D   Over age 30 at childbirth.
E   Low expectations of child.

23.8   **In childhood sexual abuse:**
A   Inappropriate sexual activity in adolescence is excluded by definition.
B   Physical contact is required for diagnosis.
C   The abuser is usually outside the family.
D   Disclosure is less likely where incest occurs.
E   Physical symptoms are rare in the abused child.

23.9   **The following symptoms in a 5-year-old are suggestive of autism:**
A   Avoidance of eye contact.
B   Poor language development.
C   Extreme reactions to change.
D   Extremely varied play.
E   Pronominal reversal.

(Answers overleaf)

23.5 A False Attachment occurs at 6 months, stranger anxiety at 10 months.
     B True
     C False There is strong preference for same-sex friends.
     D True
     E True

(Further details can be found in the *Companion to Psychiatric Studies*, pp. 652 and 654.)

23.6 A False DSM and ICD are phenomenological.
     B True
     C False ICD-10 codes mental retardation on Axis I.
     D True
     E False Mixed means a combination.

(Further details can be found in the *Companion to Psychiatric Studies*, pp. 655–656.)

23.7 A True
     B True
     C True
     D False Being young is a risk characteristic in the parent.
     E False Unrealistically high expectations of the child and his development are associated with abuse.

(Further details can be found in the *Companion to Psychiatric Studies*, p. 661.)

23.8 A False
     B False Posing for pornographic photographs, for example, need not involve physical contact.
     C False The abuser is often a member of the family.
     D True
     E False Presentation is often with physical symptoms.

(Further details can be found in the *Companion to Psychiatric Studies*, p. 662.)

23.9 A True Avoidance of eye contact is typical.
     B True
     C True
     D False Rigid stereotyped play is typical.
     E True

(Further details can be found in the *Companion to Psychiatric Studies*, p. 663.)

23.10   Childhood emotional disorders:
A   Are more common in girls than boys.
B   Most commonly present as lowered mood.
C   Occur with a prevalence of ~ 2.5%.
D   Generally have poor prognosis.
E   Rarely present with somatic symptoms.

23.11   School refusal:
A   Is also known as school phobia.
B   Is synonymous with truancy.
C   Is associated with poor school attainment.
D   Is often related to separation anxiety.
E   May be treated by behavioural means.

23.12   Enuresis:
A   Can only be diagnosed after 3 years of age.
B   Is associated with psychiatric disturbance in ~ 25% of cases.
C   Is more commonly nocturnal than diurnal.
D   Is termed secondary when there has been a 'dry period' for at least 1 year.
E   Occurs with a prevalence of ~ 5% amongst 10-year-olds.

23.13   Regarding encopresis:
A   Soiling is regarded as pathological after the fourth birthday.
B   Community prevalence is ~ 10% in 8-year old boys.
C   There is a stronger association with psychiatric illness then with enuresis.
D   Retentive encopresis is thought to be due to anxiety.
E   Discontinuous encopresis is usually due to inadequate toilet training.

23.14   Hyperkinetic disorder:
A   Is equally common in boys and girls.
B   May have mood swings as the presenting feature.
C   Occurs with a prevalence of ~ 1% in the UK.
D   Requires cross-situational overactivity for diagnosis.
E   Is at a peak between 8 and 11 years of age.

(Answers overleaf)

23.10 A **True**
    B **False** They present most commonly as anxiety.
    C **True**
    D **False** Generally the prognosis is favourable.
    E **False** They frequently present with somatic symptoms.

(Further details can be found in the *Companion to Psychiatric Studies*, p. 665.)

23.11 A **True**
    B **False** School refusal is a phobic disorder – truancy is a conduct problem.
    C **False** It is associated with good attainment.
    D **True**
    E **True**

(Further details can be found in the *Companion to Psychiatric Studies*, p. 666.)

23.12 A **False** It can be diagnosed after age 5.
    B **True**
    C **True**
    D **False** Secondary enuresis is recurrence after a 6-month 'dry period'.
    E **True**

(Further details can be found in the *Companion to Psychiatric Studies*, p. 670.)

23.13 A **True**
    B **False** It is 1–2%.
    C **True**
    D **False** It is thought to be due anger and hostility.
    E **False** Continuous encopresis is usually due to inadequate toilet training.

(Further details can be found in the *Companion to Psychiatric Studies*, p. 671.)

23.14 A **False** There is a male preponderance of 3 to 1.
    B **True**
    C **True**
    D **True**
    E **False** It is at a peak from 3 to 8 years.

(Further details can be found in the *Companion to Psychiatric Studies*, p. 672.)

24. Psychiatric disorders in adolescence

24.1 **Adolescence:**
- A   Is equivalent to puberty.
- B   Is defined as age 14–16 years.
- C   Is characterised by specific psychiatric disorders.
- D   Is a time when 25% of persons have diagnosable psychiatric disorders.
- E   Has received dedicated psychiatric services since the 1890s.

24.2 **Regarding anxiety disorder in adolescence:**
- A   School refusal is a type of social phobia.
- B   Separation anxiety is associated with school refusal.
- C   Benzodiazepines are the treatment of choice.
- D   It may present as somatic complaints.
- E   It often persists into adulthood.

24.3 **Regarding obsessive–compulsive disorder in adolescence:**
- A   Prevalence is 0.5%.
- B   Internal resistance is a diagnostic sign.
- C   It is associated with good prognosis.
- D   There is strong continuity to adulthood.
- E   Noradrenergic drugs are the treatment of choice.

24.4 **Conduct disorder in adolescence:**
- A   May persist from childhood.
- B   Is a social concept.
- C   May be diagnosed from two incidents of severe behavioural disturbance.
- D   Is of equal sex incidence.
- E   Is commoner in inner city areas.

(Answers overleaf)

24.1 A **False**
       B **False**   It is usually defined as age 12–20.
       C **False**   No psychiatric disorder is specific.
       D **True**
       E **False**   This is not true of the UK where there have only been
                      such services since the 1960s.

(Further details can be found in the *Companion to Psychiatric Studies*, pp. 683–684.)

24.2 A **False**   School refusal and school phobia are separate
                      disorders.
       B **True**
       C **False**   They may have a role but only for brief treatment as
                      they may induce dependence.
       D **True**
       E **True**   Many phobic disorders have their origin in
                      adolescence.

(Further details can be found in the *Companion to Psychiatric Studies*, p. 687.)

24.3 A **False**   Prevalence is 2%.
       B **False**   Resistance is not always present.
       C **False**   The prognosis is poor.
       D **True**
       E **False**   Serotonergic drugs and behaviour therapy are the
                      treatment of choice.

(Further details can be found in the *Companion to Psychiatric Studies*, p. 688.)

24.4 A **True**
       B **False**   Delinquency is a social concept, conduct disorder is a
                      medical diagnosis.
       C **False**   Persistent behavioural disturbance must be present.
       D **False**   It is commoner in males.
       E **True**

(Further details can be found in the *Companion to Psychiatric Studies*, pp. 690–691.)

24.5   **Symptoms of adolescent conduct disorder include:**
A   Multiple tics.
B   Fire raising.
C   Sexual dysfunction.
D   Cruelty to animals.
E   School refusal.

24.6   **Strategies for the treatment of adolescent conduct disorder include:**
A   Delayed intervention.
B   Antipsychotic medication.
C   Family therapy.
D   Star chart.
E   Imprisonment.

24.7   **Regarding alcohol abuse in adolescence:**
A   There is equal sex incidence.
B   Of 16- to 19-year-olds, 10% report themselves to be regular drinkers.
C   Half of adolescents first taste alcohol at home.
D   It is associated with an increased risk of suicide.
E   It is less prevalent than cannabis misuse.

24.8   **The following are true of adolescent substance misuse:**
A   'Crack' cocaine can cause respiratory failure.
B   'Ecstasy' is also called MMDA.
C   5% of secondary school pupils regularly abuse solvents.
D   Solvent misuse commonly produces persistent neuropsychological impairment.
E   Angel dust is also knows as PCP.

24.9   **Teenage pregnancy is commonly associated with:**
A   An abortion rate of 2 per 1000 in 16- to 19-year-olds in England and Wales.
B   Teenage fathers.
C   Increased neonatal mortality.
D   Anxiety disorder.
E   Increased psychosocial deficits in the child.

(Answers overleaf)

24.5 A False
B True
C False
D True
E False

(Further details can be found in the *Companion to Psychiatric Studies*, pp. 690–691.)

24.6 A False Early intervention is likely to be more effective.
B True Short-term use is justified.
C True Efficacy is uncertain, however.
D False Star chart is a childhood behavioural technique.
E False Imprisonment is not a treatment.

(Further details can be found in the *Companion to Psychiatric Studies*, p. 691.)

24.7 A True
B False Over 50% of this age group consider themselves to be regular drinkers.
C True
D True
E False

(Further details can be found in the *Companion to Psychiatric Studies*, p. 693.)

24.8 A True
B False It is called MDMA.
C False 5% have tried; only 0.5–1% are abusers.
D False It rarely occurs with the usual level of abuse.
E True

(Further details can be found in the *Companion to Psychiatric Studies*, pp. 693–694.)

24.9 A False The rate is 24 per 1000 in women aged 16–19 in England and Wales.
B False Most sexual partners of pregnant teenagers are in their 20s.
C True
D False There is no evidence of specific psychopathology associated.
E True

(Further details can be found in the *Companion to Psychiatric Studies*, p. 695.)

24.10 **Regarding eating disorders in adolescence:**
A   Prevalence of anorexia nervosa is 5%.
B   Boys account for 5–10% of cases of anorexia nervosa.
C   Bulimia has a prevalence of 10%.
D   Bulimia is associated with reduced body weight.
E   Family-based treatment is usually successful for anorexia nervosa.

24.11 **Regarding depressive disorder in adolescence:**
A   There is a female to male ratio of 4 : 1.
B   Promiscuity may be the presenting feature.
C   Sufferers are more likely to show psychomotor retardation than adult sufferers.
D   A positive family history is often present.
E   It is never treated with ECT.

24.12 **Regarding suicide in adolescents:**
A   It is the sixth commonest cause of death.
B   Rates for females are increasing.
C   It is associated with conduct disorder.
D   It is most common just before puberty.
E   It is often associated with suicide pacts.

24.13 **Repeated deliberate self-harm in adolescents:**
A   Occurs in 5% during the year following an initial attempt.
B   Is associated with early parental loss.
C   Is associated with living at home.
D   Is associated with poor peer relations.
E   Is associated with resolution of problems.

24.14 **In schizophrenia in adolescence:**
A   The usual age of onset of is 12.
B   The prognosis is better with younger onset.
C   Subacute sclerosing panencephalitis is a differential diagnosis.
D   First rank symptoms are easy to identify.
E   Adolescents with affective features have a poorer prognosis.

(Answers overleaf)

24.10 A **False** It is 0.5–1%.
      B **True**
      C **False** They account for only 1%.
      D **False** Body weight is usually normal.
      E **False** It is effective only in younger patients with disorders of short duration.

(Further details can be found in the *Companion to Psychiatric Studies*, p. 696.)

24.11 A **True**
      B **True**
      C **False** They are less likely.
      D **True**
      E **False** It is used in resistant severe depression.

(Further details can be found in the *Companion to Psychiatric Studies*, pp. 697–698.)

24.12 A **False** It is the third commonest cause of death after accidents and homicide.
      B **False** Rates for males are increasing.
      C **True**
      D **False** It is rare before puberty.
      E **False** These are rare.

(Further details can be found in the *Companion to Psychiatric Studies*, pp. 698–699.)

24.13 A **False** The proportion is 10%.
      B **True**
      C **False** It is associated with living away from home.
      D **True**
      E **False** Is associated with long-term problems.

(Further details can be found in the *Companion to Psychiatric Studies*, pp. 698–699.)

24.14 A **False** Onset is commonest after 15.
      B **False** There is a worse prognosis with younger onset.
      C **True**
      D **False** They may be hard to identify.
      E **False** There is a better prognosis with affective features.

(Further details can be found in the *Companion to Psychiatric Studies*, pp. 699–670.)

25. Old age psychiatry

25.1 **Regarding the over-65s in the UK:**
A   5% live in institutional care.
B   5% have major psychiatric illnesses.
C   They make up 40% of psychiatric hospital residents.
D   Half of elderly males live alone.
E   They make up approximately 30% of the population.

25.2 **Delirium in the over-65s:**
A   Occurs in 5% of admissions to medical wards.
B   Is commoner than in the under-65s.
C   Rarely fluctuates.
D   Leads to dementia in 1–2% of cases.
E   Has an identified medical cause in less than half of cases.

25.3 **The following features are more likely in delirium than in dementia:**
A   Insidious onset.
B   Stability of affect.
C   Perceptual abnormality.
D   Restlessness.
E   Visual hallucinations.

25.4 **Features of Lewy body dementia include:**
A   Eosinophilic inclusion bodies.
B   Neuroleptic insensitivity.
C   Extrapyramidal movement disorder.
D   Slow deteriorating course.
E   Mixed subcortical and cortical involvement.

25.5 **Risk factors for the development of Alzheimer's disease include:**
A   Smoking.
B   Down's syndrome.
C   APOE ε2 status.
D   Age.
E   Oestrogen exposure.

(Answers overleaf)

25.1 A **True**
B **False** 10–20% have major psychiatric illnesses.
C **False** 65% of psychiatric hospital residents are over 65.
D **False** Half of elderly females live alone; only 20% of males.
E **False** Approximately 16% of the population are over 65.

(Further details can be found in the *Companion to Psychiatric Studies*, p. 713.)

25.2 A **False** It affects 10–25% of admissions to medical wards.
B **True**
C **False** Fluctuation is characteristic.
D **False** 5% progress to dementia.
E **False** In 80–95% of cases a medical cause is identified.

(Further details can be found in the *Companion to Psychiatric Studies*, pp. 724–725.)

25.3 A **False** Abrupt onset more likely in delirium.
B **False** Lability of affect is more likely in delirium.
C **True**
D **True**
E **True**

(Further details can be found in the *Companion to Psychiatric Studies*, p. 725.)

25.4 A **True**
B **False** There is increased neuroleptic sensitivity.
C **True**
D **False** A rapidly progressive course is typical.
E **True**

(Further details can be found in the *Companion to Psychiatric Studies*, p. 729.)

25.5 A **False** Smoking has been suggested to have a protective role.
B **True**
C **False** APOE ε4 is a risk factor, APOE ε2 is protective.
D **True**
E **False** Oestrogen is thought to be protective.

(Further details can be found in the *Companion to Psychiatric Studies*, p. 728.)

25.6   **In the management of dementia in the elderly:**
A   Structural brain scans are a routine investigation.
B   Cholinesterase drugs delay cognitive decline.
C   Aspirin may be useful in vascular dementia.
D   Antipsychotic drugs may improve repetitive behaviour.
E   Antipsychotic drugs are especially useful in Lewy body dementia.

25.7   **For elderly demented patients:**
A   The Mental Health Act does not apply.
B   Relatives may give consent for incapable patients.
C   Doctors may provide consent for incapable patients.
D   Advance directives regarding treatment are legally binding in the UK.
E   Incapacity law in the UK separates financial from treatment decisions.

25.8   **Regarding functional psychosis in the elderly:**
A   It has a prevalence of 5%.
B   It is more common in males than in females.
C   There is a strong association with visual impairment.
D   First rank symptoms are present in 30%.
E   25% have premorbid paranoid and schizotypal traits.

25.9   **Regarding affective disorders beginning after age 65:**
A   They are more common in males.
B   Genetic factors are particularly important.
C   They are associated with physical illness in the majority.
D   More than 20% of cases of major depression emerge in old age.
E   There are lower rates in nursing homes.

(Answers overleaf)

25.6   **A**   **False**   Brain scans should be performed on the basis of clinical indication.
           B   **False**   Anticholinesterase drugs may delay cognitive decline.
           C   **True**   It may be useful in multi-infarct dementia.
           D   **True**   Low doses are preferable.
           E   **False**   These patients are very sensitive to these drugs.

(Further details can be found in the *Companion to Psychiatric Studies*, pp. 730–732.)

25.7   **A**   **False**   The Mental Health Act is often necessary.
           B   **False**   However, they may obtain the right to take decisions on the patient's behalf through a court.
           C   **False**   They may, however, act in the patient's best interests under common law.
           D   **False**
           E   **True**

(Further details can be found in the *Companion to Psychiatric Studies*, pp. 732–744.)

25.8   **A**   **False**   The prevalence is less than 1%.
           B   **False**   The female to male ration is between 4 : 1 and 9 : 1.
           C   **False**   There is a strong association with deafness.
           D   **True**
           E   **False**   45% have premorbid paranoid and schizotypal traits.

(Further details can be found in the *Companion to Psychiatric Studies*, p. 735.)

25.9   **A**   **False**   They are more common in females.
           B   **False**   A positive family history is less common than in earlier life.
           C   **True**   There is an association with physical illness in 60–75% cases.
           D   **False**   Less than 10% of cases of major depression emerge in old age.
           E   **False**   There are higher rates in nursing homes.

(Further details can be found in the *Companion to Psychiatric Studies*, pp. 736–737.)

25.10 **Depressive pseudodementia is more likely than dementia when the following are present:**
A   Past history of depression.
B   Hallucinations.
C   Islands of normality.
D   Agitation.
E   Exaggerated presentation of symptoms.

25.11 **Suicide in the elderly is associated with:**
A   Female gender.
B   Social isolation.
C   Hypochondriacal concerns.
D   Physical illness.
E   Poor self-care.

25.12 **Regarding deliberate self-harm in the over-65s:**
A   It is less often associated with suicidal intent.
B   It accounts for 20% of total deliberate self-harm (DSH).
C   Less than 20% are physically ill.
D   8% complete suicide within 3 years.
E   The risk factors involved differ markedly from those associated with completed suicide.

25.13 **Late-onset alcohol abuse in the elderly:**
A   Is more likely to have a positive family history than in the young.
B   Is associated with low social class.
C   Is associated with physical illness.
D   Is associated with male gender.
E   Tends to be more severe than in younger people.

25.14 **Senile squalor:**
A   Has been called Aristotle's syndrome.
B   Is associated with erotomania.
C   Is specifically associated with parietal lobe dysfunction.
D   Is rarely associated with psychiatric illness.
E   Is rarely associated with physical illness.

(Answers overleaf)

25.10 A True
      B False
      C True
      D False
      E True

(Further details can be found in the *Companion to Psychiatric Studies*, p. 737.)

25.11 A False The male rate is twice the rate for females.
      B True
      C True
      D True 35–85% cases are associated with physical illness.
      E False

(Further details can be found in the *Companion to Psychiatric Studies*, p. 739.)

25.12 A False It is more often associated with suicidal intent.
      B False It accounts for 5% of DSH.
      C False Over 60% are physically ill.
      D True
      E False Similar factors are associated.

(Further details can be found in the *Companion to Psychiatric Studies*, p. 739.)

25.13 A False A positive family history is less likely.
      B False High social class is a risk factor.
      C True
      D False Female gender is a risk factor.
      E False It tends to be milder.

(Further details can be found in the *Companion to Psychiatric Studies*, p. 741.)

25.14 A False It has been called Diogenes syndrome.
      B False The association is with syllogomania or compulsive collecting.
      C False It is associated with frontal lobe dysfunction.
      D False It is frequently associated with psychiatric illness.
      E False It is frequently associated with physical illness.

(Further details can be found in the *Companion to Psychiatric Studies*, p. 742.)

26. Suicide

26.1 Regarding suicide rates:
A Death by suicide is now nearly as frequent as that from road traffic accidents (RTAs).
B They are reliably coded throughout Europe.
C In Europe, they are lowest in the southern regions.
D They are higher in the UK than in any other European country.
E They are higher in Scotland than in England and Wales.

26.2 The following statements about suicide rates are correct:
A Suicide rates decrease as a function of age.
B Australia has the highest youth suicide rate in the industrialised world.
C In Europe the suicide rates are highest among older men.
D International differences by rank order have remained fairly constant throughout the 20th century.
E Suicide rates are falling in Japan.

26.3 The following statements about suicide methods are correct:
A Violent methods are more commonly used by the psychiatrically ill.
B Two-thirds of British male suicides result from hanging or vehicle exhaust fumes.
C One-third of British female suicides result from hanging or vehicle exhaust fumes.
D Drowning is used more often by females than males to commit suicide.
E Suicide as a result of jumping from a height is commoner among males than females.

26.1 **A** **False** The number of people dying by suicide is now significantly higher then those who die in RTAs.
     B **False** Under-reporting is the norm and practices of reporting differ. However, rates may be usefully compared between countries and over time.
     C **True** They are highest in northern countries.
     D **False** The UK has lower rates than countries which form the 'belt' of Europe, such as France through to Russia.
     E **True** Rates have been higher in Scotland since the 1970s.

(Further details can be found in the *Companion to Psychiatric Studies*, pp. 751–752.)

26.2 **A** **False** Suicide increases with increasing age.
     B **True** It is 16 per 1000 in 15- to 24-year-olds.
     C **True** Women peak at 45–64.
     D **False** Durkheim's statement in 1897 was borne out until the reversal of suicide rates in Scotland relative to England and Wales from the 1970s.
     E **True** It is no longer regarded as 'honourable'.

(Further details can be found in the *Companion to Psychiatric Studies*, pp. 752–754.)

26.3 **A** **True** Examples are hanging and shooting.
     B **True** These methods are less common in females, who use overdose more.
     C **True** These methods are more common in males.
     D **False** Drowning has no sex bias but is used more by older suicides.
     E **False** Jumping from a height has no sex bias but is commoner in younger suicides.

(Further details can be found in the *Companion to Psychiatric Studies*, p. 754.)

26.4   **The following statements about subjects who survived after throwing themselves in front of London Underground trains are correct:**

A   A minority of such patients have severe mental illness.
B   Few of these persons were currently receiving psychiatric treatment.
C   The suicide attempt was generally unplanned.
D   Subjects often travelled long distances to carry out such a suicide attempt.
E   This method was unrelated to its perceived dangerousness.

26.5   **The following statements about attempts to reduce suicide rates are correct:**

A   Domestic gas detoxification in the UK resulted in a one-third reduction of the suicide rate in the 1960s.
B   States of the USA with the lowest circulation of firearm magazines have the lowest suicide rates.
C   States of the USA with the lowest rates of firearm-related suicides have a compensatory increase in the use of other methods.
D   The newer antidepressant drugs are less toxic.
E   It has been estimated that up to 5000 lives per year in Britain may be saved by using selective serotonin reuptake inhibitors (SSRIs) rather than tricyclic drugs as first-line treatment for depression.

26.6   **In young males, suicide:**

A   Is becoming more common.
B   Is commoner in subjects who live with their parents.
C   Is associated with a past history of psychiatric admission.
D   Is associated with increasing rates of severe mental illness in young adults.
E   Rates are rising particularly in the 25- to 34-year age group.

26.7   **Biological variables implicated in deliberate self-harm (DSH) include:**

A   5-hydroxytryptamine (5-HT).
B   Cholesterol.
C   Tryptophan.
D   Thyroxine.
E   Homovanillic acid (HVA).

(Answers overleaf)

26.4   A   **False**   The majority have mental illness.
     B   **False**   Most were receiving treatment.
     C   **True**   Often little or no planning is involved.
     D   **False**   The ready availability of this method was an important factor in its choice.
     E   **False**   It was chosen because it was perceived as dangerous.

(Further details can be found in the *Companion to Psychiatric Studies*, p. 754.)

26.5   A   **True**   Putting one's head in the gas oven was a common method of suicide.
     B   **True**   Firearms are a common method of suicide in the USA.
     C   **False**   There appears to be almost no compensatory increase in other methods.
     D   **True**   Although it is debatable whether this translates to a reduced suicide rate.
     E   **False**   The estimate is 450 and this figure does not take possible method substitution into account.

(Further details can be found in the *Companion to Psychiatric Studies*, pp. 754–755.)

26.6   A   **True**   There has been a major increase.
     B   **True**   Although it appears paradoxical.
     C   **True**   This is in keeping with the association of suicide with mental illness.
     D   **False**   There is little evidence that severe mental illness has increased among young adults.
     E   **False**   Rather, rates are rising in the 15- to 24-year age group.

(Further details can be found in the *Companion to Psychiatric Studies*, pp. 755–756.)

26.7   A   **True**   Lower 5-HT is associated with more serious attempts.
     B   **True**   Low cholesterol is found following DSH.
     C   **True**   There is some evidence in violent offenders.
     D   **False**   There is no evidence for this.
     E   **True**   Urinary and cerebrospinal fluid levels of HVA are reduced in DSH.

(Further details can be found in the *Companion to Psychiatric Studies*, p. 758.)

26.8 **The following statements about suicide are correct:**

A   The majority of persons committing suicide have a psychiatric disorder.

B   Alcohol dependence is the commonest mental disorder in patients who kill themselves.

C   Suicide is rare among those with good physical and mental health.

D   In Taiwan there is a weaker association between psychiatric disorder and suicide than in the West.

E   More than 20% of suicides are suffering from schizophrenia.

26.9 **Clinical correlates of suicide in persons with major depression include:**

A   Self-neglect.

B   Impaired concentration.

C   Psychotic symptoms.

D   A history of deliberate self-harm.

E   Insomnia.

26.10 **Long-term predictors of suicide include:**

A   Anhedonia.

B   Alcohol abuse.

C   Somatisation.

D   A history of deliberate self-harm.

F   Anxiety

26.11 **The main correlates of suicide in persons with schizophrenia are:**

A   Chronic, unremitting illness.

B   Good insight.

C   Young males.

D   A past history of depression.

E   A past history of deliberate self-harm.

(Answers overleaf)

26.8   A   **True**   Over 90% has been reported.
         B   **False**   Depression is the commonest diagnosis (70%); alcohol dependence is the second most common (15%).
         C   **True**   There is a strong association with illness, both medical and psychiatric.
         D   **False**   Similar patterns are reported in eastern and western cultures.
         E   **False**   Reported rates are less than 5% of all suicides, although suicide is a common cause of death in schizophrenia.

(Further details can be found in the *Companion to Psychiatric Studies*, p. 756.)

26.9   A   **True**
         B   **True**
         C   **False**   Recent studies have found no major differences between psychotic and non-psychotic depressives.
         D   **True**
         E   **True**

(Further details can be found in the *Companion to Psychiatric Studies*, p. 758.)

26.10   A   **False**   It is a short-term predictor.
         B   **False**   It is a short-term predictor.
         C   **False**   There is no evidence for this.
         D   **True**
         E   **False**   It is a short-term predictor.

(Further details can be found in the *Companion to Psychiatric Studies*, p. 758.)

26.11   A   **False**   Relapsing pattern of illness is a major correlate.
         B   **True**   Such patients are probably at greater risk.
         C   **True**
         D   **True**
         E   **True**

(Further details can be found in the *Companion to Psychiatric Studies*, p. 760.)

26.12 **The following statements about suicide in alcoholic patients are correct:**
A   The lifetime risk of suicide in alcoholics is 10%.
B   The mean age at suicide is 35 years.
C   Two-thirds of alcoholic suicides have a past history of deliberate self-harm.
D   It usually occurs when the patient is abstinent.
E   Male alcoholics have a suicide rate twice that of female alcoholics.

26.13 **The following statements about deliberate self-harm (DSH) are correct:**
A   DSH rates mirror trends in suicide rates.
B   Persons committing DSH have 1000 times the general population's risk of suicide.
C   The age at which people first deliberately harm themselves is decreasing.
D   Almost all cases of DSH are admitted to hospital.
E   DSH is a major risk factor for subsequent suicide.

26.14 **The following statements about deliberate self-harm (DSH) are true:**
A   Large multicentre randomised controlled trials have shown that cognitive–behavioural therapy significantly reduces the rate of suicide after DSH.
B   Patients admitted with DSH are no more likely to die from causes other than suicide than the general population.
C   A contact card scheme for DSH patients has been shown to reduce the repeat DSH admission rate.
D   Approximately 50% of DSH admissions involve repeaters.
E   15% of patients committing DSH will repeat an episode of DSH within the following year.

(Answers overleaf)

26.12   **A**   **False**   The risk is 2% for those with a history of outpatient treatment; it is 3% for those with a history of inpatient treatment.
      B   **False**   The mean age is 47 years.
      C   **False**   One-third have a history of deliberate self-harm.
      D   **False**   It usually occurs when the patient is drinking.
      E   **True**

(Further details can be found in the *Companion to Psychiatric Studies*, p. 761.)

26.13   **A**   **True**
      B   **False**   The risk is 100 times greater than that of the general population.
      C   **True**
      D   **False**   Population surveys suggest that many are not admitted.
      E   **True**   10–14% of DSH patients eventually die by suicide.

(Further details can be found in the *Companion to Psychiatric Studies*, pp. 765–766.)

26.14   **A**   **False**   Large trials would be required but have not been performed.
      B   **False**   10-year follow-up shows an increased rate from disease and accidents.
      C   **True**   The Bristol Green Card Scheme reduced this by 50%.
      D   **True**
      E   **True**

(Further details can be found in the *Companion to Psychiatric Studies*, pp. 773–774.)

27. Liaison psychiatry

27.1   **The most common psychiatric disorders encountered in medical outpatients are:**
A   Depression and anxiety.
B   Delirium.
C   Alcohol problems.
D   Somatoform disorders.
E   Psychosis.

27.2   **Psychiatric comorbidity in medical patients is associated with:**
A   Poorer medical outcomes.
B   Less disability.
C   A lower consumption of general medical resources.
D   Presentation often being with somatic complaints.
E   Doctors finding their patients difficult to help.

27.3   **The following statements about somatic presentations are correct:**
A   Unexplained somatic complaints imply a diagnosis of somatoform disorder.
B   Somatoform disorder can only be diagnosed in patients with no medical disease.
C   A diagnoses of chronic fatigue syndrome excludes a diagnosis of somatoform disorder.
D   The majority of unexplained somatic symptoms are mild and transient.
E   The somatic symptoms of one-third of all cardiology outpatients remain medically unexplained at the time of discharge.

(Answers overleaf)

27.1 A **True**   Approximately 20% are cases.
       B **False** It is commonly seen in medical and surgical inpatients.
       C **True**   Prevalence depends on threshold.
       D **True**   5–20% are cases.
       E **False** It is very rare in this setting.

(Further details can be found in the *Companion to Psychiatric Studies*, p. 787.)

27.2 A **True**   There is evidence in stroke and myocardial infarction.
       B **False** Depression magnifies the disability associated with the medical condition.
       C **False** It is associated with increased utilisation of medical resources.
       D **True**   Presentation with obvious depressed mood is less common than in psychiatric settings.
       E **True**   There is a strong association with doctors' perception of difficulty.

(Further details can be found in the *Companion to Psychiatric Studies*, p. 787.)

27.3 A **False** A diagnosis of depressive or anxiety disorder is more common.
       B **False** Patients may have both a medical condition and a somatoform disorder.
       C **False** Functional syndromes such as chronic fatigue syndrome are simply alternative (medical) labels for (psychiatric) somatoform disorders.
       D **True**   Most symptoms identified in population surveys do not lead to medical consultation.
       E **True**   This is true of most medical specialties.

(Further details can be found in the *Companion to Psychiatric Studies*, p. 789.)

27.4   **The following statements about the classification of psychiatric disorders are correct:**

A   Comorbid medical conditions are recorded on Axis IV of DSM-IV.

B   The ICD-10 classification requires the recording of comorbid medical conditions.

C   'Organic mental disorder' is a DSM-IV diagnosis.

D   Current classifications offer two main ways of coding comorbidity.

E   Depression and anxiety in medical patients are best recorded as 'mental disorders due to a general medical condition'.

27.5   **The following medical conditions have been shown to probably cause depression by a direct biological mechanism:**

A   Stroke.

B   Pancreatitis.

C   Multiple sclerosis.

D   Hypothyroidism.

E   Hyperthyroidism.

27.6   **Medical conditions are more likely to cause depression when:**

A   The patient has no previous history of depression.

B   They are infectious.

C   They are disfiguring.

D   They cause disability.

E   They are potentially fatal.

(Answers overleaf)

27.4   A   **False**   They are recorded on Axis III.
        B   **True**   This is included in the instruction for use, although ICD-10 is not fully multiaxial like DSM-IV.
        C   **False**   This is an ICD-10 category.
        D   **True**   Either the medical diagnosis is coded separately using a multiaxial approach, or it is coded as a consequence of the medical condition as an 'organic mental disorder' (ICD) or 'mental disorder due to a medical condition' (DSM).
        E   **False**   This implies that the medical condition has caused the mental disorder – this is usually difficult to establish and it is therefore generally better to use the multiaxial method.

(Further details can be found in the *Companion to Psychiatric Studies*, p. 790.)

27.5   A   **True**   But it is controversial whether a specific part of the brain is involved.
        B   **False**   There is no evidence for this (but pancreatic cancer probably can).
        C   **True**   There is some evidence for this.
        D   **True**   There is some evidence for this.
        E   **False**   There is no evidence for this (it is more likely to mimic an anxiety state).

(Further details can be found in the *Companion to Psychiatric Studies*, p. 792.)

27.6   A   **False**   Previous history of depression is a major risk factor.
        B   **False**   There is no evidence for this.
        C   **True**   There is loss of appearance/previous attractiveness.
        D   **True**   There is loss of previous function/activities.
        E   **True**   There is loss of future/plans.

Note: Personal vulnerability is especially important. (Further details can be found in the *Companion to Psychiatric Studies*, p. 792.)

27.7 Screening questionnaires for detecting psychiatric morbidity in medically ill patients include the:
A PSE.
B HAD.
C PRIME MD.
D AUDIT.
E MMSE.

27.8 In non-psychiatric medical settings, major depression:
A Occurs in approximately 15% of patients in primary care.
B Occurs in 5–10% of medical outpatients.
C Occurs in 40–50% of medical inpatients.
D Is the most common form of depression in the chronically medically ill.
E When comorbid with a medical condition does not respond to antidepressant drug treatment.

27.9 In non-psychiatric medical settings, panic disorder:
A Is a common accompaniment of hypochondriasis.
B Is a common cause of non-cardiac chest pain.
C Is a common cause of chronic persistent pain.
D Is a particular problem for patients with insulin dependent diabetes mellitus.
E Is associated with increased use of psychiatric but not non-psychiatric medical services.

27.10 Somatisation disorder:
A Is also known as Birket's syndrome.
B May be diagnosed in 1–4% of the general population.
C May be diagnosed in 10–20% of medical patients.
D Is strongly associated with personality disorder.
E Has a good prognosis.

(Answers overleaf)

27.7 A False It is a detailed psychiatric interview.
      B True   It is designed to screen for depression and anxiety in
                medical patients.
      C False It is a brief psychiatric interview.
      D True   It is an alcohol misuse screening questionnaire.
      E True   It is a brief interview to screen for cognitive
                impairment.

(Further details can be found in the *Companion to Psychiatric Studies*, p. 794.)

27.8 A False Prevalence is approximately 5%.
      B True   The precise rate depends on method of diagnosis and
                population sampled.
      C False 10–20% is the range commonly reported.
      D False Milder forms such as dysthymia are more prevalent.
      E False A recent systematic review confirms their
                effectiveness in comorbid depression.

(Further details can be found in the *Companion to Psychiatric Studies*, p. 796.)

27.9 A True   Both share unexplained symptoms, anxiety and fear
                of dying.
      B True   Presumably, this is via the mechanism of
                hyperventilation.
      C False Panic symptoms are episodic.
      D False Specific (needle) phobia is more likely to be a
                particular problem.
      E False Patients with panic are high utilisers of both.

(Further details can be found in the *Companion to Psychiatric Studies*, pp. 796–797.)

27.10 A False It is also known as Briquet's syndrome after a French
                physician.
      B True   Prevalence depends on the definition used and
                sampling.
      C True   Prevalence depends on the definition used and
                sampling.
      D True   In fact it has been argued that it is better regarded as
                a personality disorder.
      E False The prognosis is very poor.

(Further details can be found in the *Companion to Psychiatric Studies*, pp. 797–798.)

27.11 **The following statements regarding conversion disorder are correct:**
A   The prognosis for acute conversion symptoms is good.
B   At long-term follow-up most patients turn out to have a neurological disease.
C   It is a form of factitious disorder.
D   The form of the symptoms is influenced by the personal experience of the patient.
E   Conversion disorder is no longer encountered in specialist medical practice.

27.12 **Chronic medically unexplained fatigue:**
A   Is best coded as undifferentiated somatoform disorder in ICD-10.
B   Is strongly associated with current depressive disorders.
C   Is not associated with previous depressive disorders.
D   Io known as neurasthenia in the DSM-IV classification.
E   Is the core symptom of the chronic fatigue syndrome.

27.13 **The following statements about hypochondriasis are correct:**
A   Anxiety symptoms are common in patients with hypochondriasis.
B   It is usually delusional.
C   Hypochondriacal states are rarely transient.
D   Established hypochondriasis affects approximately 5% of medical outpatients.
E   Hypochondriasis is best treated by repeated reassurance.

(Answers overleaf)

27.11 A True Most are related to acute stressors and transient.
       B False A much quoted study suggesting this (Slater) has been refuted by more recent research.
       C False In factitious disorder, symptoms are intentionally produced – conversion is unconscious.
       D True For example, symptoms may be modelled on the illness of a sick parent.
       E False Conversion is frequently seen in specialist practice, especially neurology, although perhaps less commonly than 100 years ago.

(Further details can be found in the *Companion to Psychiatric Studies*, p. 798.)

27.12 A False It is diagnosed as neurasthenia in ICD-10, undifferentiated somatoform disorder in DSM-IV.
       B True 50% or more of patients have major depression in specialist clinics.
       C False There is a strong association also with previous major depressive disorder.
       D False It is termed undifferentiated somatoform disorder in DSM-IV.
       E True Chronic fatigue syndrome is the functional medical syndrome that is the approximate equivalent of the psychiatric syndrome of neurasthenia.

(Further details can be found in the *Companion to Psychiatric Studies*, p. 798.)

27.13 A True Some regard hypochondriasis as an anxiety disorder.
       B False It is rarely delusional in general medical populations.
       C False Transient hypochondriasis is common, e.g. in medical students.
       D True Although minor hypochondriacal states are more common.
       E False Repeated reassurance is a perpetuating factor.

(Further details can be found in the *Companion to Psychiatric Studies*, pp. 798.)

27.14 **The following statements about substance misuse are correct:**

A A history of substance misuse is rare amongst medical patients.

B 20% of male medical admissions are problem drinkers.

C Drug misusers represent approximately 20% of attendees at inner city casualty departments.

D Giving problem drinkers advice on intake has little effect.

E The misuse of drugs other than alcohol has now overtaken alcohol as the commonest substance abuse disorder encountered in medical settings.

(Answers overleaf)

27.14   A   **False**   If alcohol misuse is included, it occurs in
                        approximately 20% of medical admissions.
        B   **True**   In some specialties (e.g. gastroenterology) it may be
                        higher.
        C   **True**   It is a major problem in inner cities.
        D   **False**   It has been shown to have useful effect.
        E   **False**   Alcohol is still the commonest, although the misuse
                        of other drugs is an increasing problem.

(Further details can be found in the *Companion to Psychiatric
Studies*, p. 800.)

28. Forensic psychiatry

28.1 **Research into the relationship between genetic factors and crime has revealed:**

A   A concordance for criminality up to six times greater in monozygotic twins that dizygotic twins.

B   A greater correlation in criminal behaviour between adopted children and their biological parents than their adoptive parents.

C   A strong correlation between an extra Y chromosome and offending.

D   A stronger genetic link for property crime compared to violent crime.

E   A modest correlation between genetic factors and crime.

28.2 **Research into the relationship between intelligence and crime has revealed:**

A   No evidence that below average intelligence is associated with crime.

B   That offenders with below average intelligence are more likely to be caught

C   That below average intelligence is associated with certain criminal behaviour.

D   Suspected offenders with mild learning disability are no more suggestible than suspected offenders of average intelligence at police interview.

E   There is a strong relationship between sexual offending and intellectual impairment.

28.1 A **True**
        B **True**
        C **False**   This is a false finding from the 1960s.
        D **True**
        E **True**

(Further details can be found in the *Companion to Psychiatric Studies*, pp. 807–808.)

28.2 A **False**   A link between low intelligence and delinquency is well established.
        B **False**
        C **True**   See A above.
        D **False**
        E **False**   However, an American study has reported an association between low IQ, murder and suffering sexual abuse.

(Further details can be found in the *Companion to Psychiatric Studies*, p. 808.)

28.3   Within a prison population:

A   Psychotic illness in remand prisoners occurs at a similar rate compared to that in the general population.

B   Rates of mental illness are higher in sentenced prisoners compared to remand prisoners.

C   Personality disorder is more common in female prisoners compared to male prisoners.

D   Substance abuse is more common in female prisoners compared to male prisoners.

E   Psychotic illness is more common in female prisoners compared to male prisoners.

28.4   Learning disability is strongly associated with:

A   Arson.

B   Sexual offences.

C   Violent offences.

D   Public order offences.

E   Paedophilia.

28.5   Factitious illness by proxy:

A   Most commonly involves mothers feigning symptoms in their children.

B   Has been associated with serial killings in the UK.

C   Is associated with schizophrenia.

D   Is associated with borderline personality disorder.

E   Is associated with eating disorder.

28.6   Recidivism amongst discharged mentally disordered offenders is associated with:

A   A diagnosis of schizophrenia.

B   A diagnosis of psychopathic disorder.

C   A longer period of detention.

D   An index offence of homicide.

E   Younger age.

(Answers overleaf)

28.3 A **False**   2–5% of remanded prisoners are psychotic.
      B **False**   Ill offenders are often diverted.
      C **True**
      D **True**
      E **False**

(Further details can be found in the *Companion to Psychiatric Studies*, pp. 809–810.)

28.4 A **False**   The rate of offending was overestimated from
                     hospital-based cohorts.
      B **False**   See A above.
      C **True**   They are increased by about 12 times in female and
                     eight times in male cases.
      D **False**   Property offending predominates.
      E **False**   See A above.

(Further details can be found in the *Companion to Psychiatric Studies*, pp. 811–813.)

28.5 A **True**
      B **True**   They have been carried out by health care workers.
      C **False**   The main psychiatric associations are with
                     personality, somatisation, affective and eating
                     disorders.
      D **True**
      E **True**

(Further details can be found in the *Companion to Psychiatric Studies*, p. 814.)

28.6 A **False**   A major psychiatric diagnosis is largely irrelevant.
      B **True**
      C **True**
      D **False**   Property offenders are more likely to reoffend.
      E **True**

(Further details can be found in the *Companion to Psychiatric Studies*, p. 815.)

28.7   Indecent exposure:

A   Was classically described by De Sade in the 19th century.

B   Rarely involves physical assault.

C   Rarely is sexually exciting to the perpetrator.

D   Commonly is associated with mental illness.

E   Is associated with more serious risk of future offending when there is a history of childhood conduct disorder.

28.8   Regarding arson:

A   There are about 30 000 episodes of arson in England and Wales per year.

B   The 'clear-up' rate is amongst the lowest for any crime.

C   It is linked in classical psychodynamic theory to the oral–anal stage of development.

D   Female arsonists are more likely to have a history of sexual abuse than other female prisoners.

E   It is strongly associated with the presence of a learning disability.

28.9   Government policy on the services for mentally disordered offenders in England, Wales and Scotland:

A   Supports the development of special hospitals as centres of excellence.

B   Is that there should be at no greater level of security than is justified.

C   Is that care should be provided as close as possible to the mentally disordered offender's home.

D   Recommends the development of therapeutic communities for personality disordered offenders in prison.

E   Recommends a massive expansion in the provision of medium security beds.

28.10   The following factors may affect the mens rea for a particular crime (in England, Wales and Scotland):

A   Age.

B   Mental disorder.

C   Non-insane automatism.

D   Acute confusion.

E   Voluntary intoxication.

(Answers overleaf)

28.7 **A** **False** Exhibitionists were classically described by Lasègue in 1877.

 B **True**

 C **False** The perpetrator is sexually excited and tends to masturbate later.

 D **False**

 E **True**

(Further details can be found in the *Companion to Psychiatric Studies*, p. 818.)

28.8 **A** **True**

 B **True** It is about 16%.

 C **False** Freud linked arson and sexual disorder but there is no evidence for this.

 D **False** The rates are the same.

 E **False** Arson and learning disability are only associated in secure hospital populations.

(Further details can be found in the *Companion to Psychiatric Studies*, pp. 819–820.)

28.9 **A** **False** A range of inpatient options is required.

 B **True**

 C **True**

 D **False**

 E **True**

(Further details can be found in the *Companion to Psychiatric Studies*, p. 827.)

28.10 **A** **True** Children are generally not held to be criminally responsible.

 B **True**

 C **True**

 D **True**

 E **False** Voluntary intoxication by itself does not constitute a defence.

(Further details can be found in the *Companion to Psychiatric Studies*, p. 823.)

28.11   Infanticide (England and Wales):

A   Is the offence committed when a child less than 1 year old is unlawfully killed by his or her parent with malice aforethought.

B   Can be extended to children of over 12 months if the mother is still breastfeeding.

C   Has the same range of psychiatric disposals available to the Court as are available for a conviction of manslaughter.

D   Was thought to be associated with milk fever.

E   Occurs at a rate of 25 per year in England and Wales.

28.12   Regarding psychiatric disposals from court (England, Wales and Scotland):

A   They usually take place after conviction.

B   Hospital orders are usually limited in time to the length of time the mentally disordered offender would have served in prison as a tariff for the offence.

C   They cannot be applied after a conviction for murder.

D   Hospital orders are usually subject to special restrictions regarding hospital transfer and discharge.

E   Hospital orders rely on a bed being available within a reasonable time period after which the mentally disordered offender may be sent to prison.

28.13   Automatism (England, Wales and Scotland):

A   Is a clinical concept.

B   Can be defined as an automatic behaviour.

C   May rarely be under voluntary control.

D   When secondary to a disease of the mind is always termed insane automatism.

E   When secondary to epileptic seizure may be termed non-insane automatism.

28.14   Fitness to plead (England, Wales and Scotland):

A   Is determined by psychiatric expert opinion.

B   Requires the ability to distinguish between a plea of guilty and not guilty.

C   If found to be absent there is always a trial of the facts to establish actus rea.

D   If found to be absent an accused is detained until he or she becomes fit to plead.

E   Rarely is said to be impaired because the accused has amnesia for the alleged offence.

(Answers overleaf)

28.11 **A** **False** A legal infanticide verdict requires a disturbance of mind.
B **False** The child must be aged less than 12 months.
C **True**
D **True** It can still be attributed to the effects of lactation.
E **False** There are fewer than five per year.

(Further details can be found in the *Companion to Psychiatric Studies*, p. 825.)

28.12 **A** **True**
B **False**
C **True**
D **False** The responsible medical officer can arrange transfer/discharge as he or she sees fit.
E **True**

(Further details can be found in the *Companion to Psychiatric Studies*, pp. 825–826.)

28.13 **A** **False** It is a legal concept.
B **False** Automatic behaviour is a clinical concept.
C **False** It is by definition involuntary.
D **True**
E **False** This is an insane automatism.

(Further details can be found in the *Companion to Psychiatric Studies*, p. 824.)

28.14 **A** **False** It is a matter for a jury in a crown court (England) after hearing psychiatric evidence.
B **True**
C **True** This was introduced in the 1991 Act in England and is paralleled in Scottish legislation.
D **False** See C above.
E **False** Mental state at the time of the offence is irrelevant.

(Further details can be found in the *Companion to Psychiatric Studies*, p. 822.)

29. Ethics

29.1 **In 1981 ethical guidance from the BMA included advice on:**
A   Private fees.
B   Torture.
C   Adultery with patients.
D   Advertising.
E   Capital punishment.

29.2 **The Hippocratic Oath:**
A   Has its origins in the Scottish Enlightenment.
B   Prohibits abortion.
C   Prohibits adultery with patients.
D   Allows euthanasia in exceptional circumstances.
E   Allows breach of confidentiality in exceptional circumstances.

29.3 **Clear examples of abusive psychiatric practice include:**
A   Euthanasia for those deemed Lebensunwertes leben.
B   The diagnosis of sluggish schizophrenia.
C   ECT for children.
D   Psychiatric care in Japan.
E   Psychiatric care on the Greek island of Leros.

29.4 **The contractarian model of the doctor–patient relationship:**
A   Rejects paternalism.
B   Requires the patient to have detailed knowledge of his disease and proposed treatment to reduce asymmetry of knowledge between a patient and doctor.
C   Acknowledges that there will always be asymmetry of power between doctor and patient.
D   Cannot justify non-consental hospital detention.
E   Cannot apply to situations where the patient lacks the capacity to choose treatment options.

(Answers overleaf)

29.1 A **True** 'Any undisclosed division of professional fees is unethical'.

B **False**

C **True** The advice was to avoid adultery (at least with one's patients).

D **True**

E **False**

(Further details can be found in the *Companion to Psychiatric Studies*, p. 834.)

29.2 A **False** Hippocrates lived in Ancient Greece.

B **True**

C **True**

D **False** Euthanasia was absolutely prohibited.

E **False**

(Further details can be found in the *Companion to Psychiatric Studies*, p. 834.)

29.3 A **True** The Nazi culling of those 'lives unworthy of life' included schizophrenics and epileptics.

B **True** The diagnosis medicalised politically unacceptable behaviour.

C **False**

D **False** There is continuing concern about but no clear current evidence of abuse in Japan.

E **True** Patients were just dumped there.

(Further details can be found in the *Companion to Psychiatric Studies*, p. 836.)

29.4 A **True**

B **False** There is unavoidable asymmetry of knowledge but no asymmetry of power.

C **False** See B above.

D **True** Paternalism justifies involuntary admission.

E **True** As is often the case in psychiatry.

(Further details can be found in the *Companion to Psychiatric Studies*, p. 837.)

29.5   **Thomas Szasz:**

   A   Has argued from a philosophical perspective that mental illness is a valid concept.

   B   Is the author of *The Divided Self*.

   C   Is a professor of psychiatry.

   D   Is a leading anti-psychiatrist.

   E   Identifies psychiatrists who treat non-consentially as frauds and agents of social control.

29.6   **R D Laing:**

   A   Saw schizophrenia as a sane response to an insane society.

   B   Was a professor of sociology.

   C   Is the author of *Asylums*.

   D   Is the author of *The Myth of Mental Illness*.

   E   Has been supported in recent years by the writings of Fulford.

29.7   **Non-maleficence and beneficence:**

   A   Is an ethical principle dating from the Renaissance.

   B   Has its origins in the epithet *primum non nocere* (first – or above all – do no harm).

   C   Is consistent with balancing the burdens and benefits of any treatment option to help decide a course of action.

   D   Underpins the contractarian view of doctor–patient relationships.

   E   Underpins the teleological view of morality.

29.8   **Confidentiality between a doctor and a patient as described in the Hippocratic Oath:**

   A   Is absolute.

   B   Can be broken in extreme circumstances to avoid harm to others.

   C   Can be broken to avoid an epidemic.

   D   Can be broken to avoid or solve a case of murder.

   E   Can be broken when an individual lacks the ability to consent to voluntary disclosure.

(Answers overleaf)

29.5 A **False**   He thinks it is an invalid concept.
      B **False**   R D Laing wrote *The Divided Self.*
      C **True**
      D **True**
      E **True**

(Further details can be found in the *Companion to Psychiatric Studies*, p. 837.)

29.6 A **True**
      B **False**   Laing was a psychiatrist.
      C **False**   Goffman wrote *Asylums.*
      D **False**   Szasz wrote *The Myth of Mental Illness.*
      E **False**   Fulford criticises both Laing and Szasz.

(Further details can be found in the *Companion to Psychiatric Studies*, p. 837.)

29.7 A **False**   It has an ancient origin.
      B **True**
      C **True**   Because it is often not possible to avoid all harm.
      D **True**   In the contractarian/deontological model, autonomy is paramount and beneficence derivative but both affect doctor–patient relations.
      E **False**   Teleology generates beneficence rather than the other way round.

(Further details can be found in the *Companion to Psychiatric Studies*, p. 838.)

29.8 A **True**
      B **False**
      C **False**
      D **False**
      E **False**

As the Hippocratic Oath is absolute it can never be broken; in clinical practice it is therefore seen as important but relative, contingent and overridable. (Further details can be found in the *Companion to Psychiatric Studies*, pp. 840–841.)

29.9   **Regarding the Tarasoff Judgement:**
A   It is binding in courts in England and Wales.
B   It arose from the murder of Podder by Tarasoff.
C   It arose because a murder victim's parents sued the perpetrator's psychotherapist for not disclosing confidential information.
D   In this case the psychotherapist failed to disclose confidential information to the police which may have prevented a murder.
E   The court ruled that clinicians had a legal duty to warn third parties who were at risk from their patients.

29.10   **A doctor examining a patient without consent:**
A   May be charged with assault.
B   May have committed a tort.
C   May be justified in the action by common law.
D   May be justified in the action by the patient's lack of capacity to consent.
E   Can ignore any advance directive.

29.11   **Implicit consent requires:**
A   Full explanation of the proposed examination or procedure.
B   Explanation of the proposed examination or procedure to the patient's satisfaction.
C   The patient to sign a declaration that the examination or procedure has been explained to him and that he consents to it.
D   Careful documentation in the notes.
E   Only verbal consent from the patient.

29.12   **The Sidaway case:**
A   Involved a man undergoing ECT.
B   Involved a woman undergoing spinal surgery.
C   Ruled that a 1% chance of a serious complication must be revealed to a patient undergoing a procedure prior to consent.
D   Ruled that practitioners must follow the standards defined by a body of medical expertise.
E   Ruled that patients must be given full information about any proposed procedure.

(Answers overleaf)

29.9 A **False** It was a Californian case and is not binding in the UK.
B **False** Podder murdered Tarasoff.
C **True** Tarasoff's parents sued.
D **False** The psychotherapist warned the police but not Tarasoff.
E **True**

(Further details can be found in the *Companion to Psychiatric Studies*, pp. 840–841.)

29.10 A **True**
B **True** A tort is a civil wrong.
C **True**
D **True**
E **False**

(Further details can be found in the *Companion to Psychiatric Studies*, p. 841.)

29.11 A **False**
B **False**
C **False**
D **False**
E **False**

Implicit or explicit consent requires the patient to be informed, competent and free of duress to be valid. (Further details can be found in the *Companion to Psychiatric Studies*, p. 841.)

29.12 A **False**
B **True**
C **False** The ruling was that doctors had no duty to divulge risks of 1%.
D **False** It followed this general principle rather than created it.
E **False**

(Further details can be found in the *Companion to Psychiatric Studies*, p. 842.)

29.13 **An advance directive:**

A Must be fully adhered to by doctors in the UK.

B Can be changed by a competent individual at any time.

C If not followed, would leave the medical practitioner open to criminal prosecution.

D Can be changed by a nominated proxy.

E Can be changed by a solicitor with enduring power of attorney.

29.14 **Compulsory treatment:**

A Cannot be justified on teleological grounds.

B Cannot be justified on deontological grounds.

C Is consistent with a contractual approach.

D Can be justified by the principle of autonomy.

E Can be justified by the principle of beneficence and non-maleficence.

(Answers overleaf)

29.13 A False Whether they are legally binding is still debated.
       B True
       C True
       D False
       E False

(Further details can be found in the *Companion to Psychiatric Studies*, pp. 843–844.)

29.14 A False A teleologist could justify compulsion where others have to judge interests.
       B False A deontologist could justify compulsion to restore autonomy.
       C False It is paternalistic.
       D False Autonomy is temporarily overridden.
       E True Acting in what psychiatrists judge to be the patient's best interests and built in safeguards for compulsion are in accordance with the principles of beneficence and non-maleficence respectively.

(Further details can be found in the *Companion to Psychiatric Studies*, p. 845.)

30. Psychological therapies

30.1 **The following are classified as supportive psychotherapy:**
- A Brief dynamic therapy.
- B Cognitive therapy.
- C Reassurance.
- D Milieu therapy.
- E Ventilation.

30.2 **Psychological 'defence mechanisms':**
- A Are only used by persons with neurosis.
- B Are conscious attempts to manage distress.
- C May be adaptive.
- D Were described by Skinner.
- E Allow for stressful situations to be coped with by distorting reality.

30.3 **The following are recognised defence mechanisms:**
- A Repression.
- B Regression.
- C Retaliation.
- D Rationalisation.
- E Reaction formation.

30.4 **Transference refers to:**
- A Feelings experienced by the patient towards the therapist originating from past experiences.
- B Feelings experienced by the therapist towards the patient originating from the therapist's past experiences.
- C A process regarded by Freud as only occurring during analysis.
- D The process by which the patient challenges negative thoughts.
- E A process not mentioned during analysis.

(Answers overleaf)

30.1   A   **False**   This is a type of 'reconstructive' therapy.
      B   **False**   This is classified as re-educative.
      C   **True**
      D   **True**
      E   **True**

(Further details can be found in the *Companion to Psychiatric Studies*, p. 847.)

30.2   A   **False**   They are reported to be universal.
      B   **False**   They are reportedly unconscious.
      C   **True**   There is some evidence of better outcome, e.g. with denial.
      D   **False**   They were described by Freud.
      E   **True**   An example is the use of denial.

(Further details can be found in the *Companion to Psychiatric Studies*, p. 848.)

30.3   A   **True**
      B   **True**
      C   **False**
      D   **True**
      E   **True**

Note: True denial, projection, displacement, undoing, turning against the self, sublimation and compensation are other defence mechanisms. Retaliation is not a defence mechanism. (Further details can be found in the *Companion to Psychiatric Studies*, p. 849.)

30.4   A   **True**
      B   **False**   This is countertransference.
      C   **False**   Such feelings may be strong in analysis but Freud regarded them as occurring in most relationships.
      D   **False**   This is a cognitive therapy technique.
      E   **False**   Interpretation of the transference is a central part of therapy.

(Further details can be found in the *Companion to Psychiatric Studies*, p. 850.)

30.5   **According to Freud's structural theory of mind, the 'id':**
   A   Is entirely unconscious.
   B   Represents conscious sense of self.
   C   Is located in the pineal gland.
   D   Is the locus of unconscious motives and repressed memories.
   E   Is experienced as if it were an external force.

30.6   **According to Freud's structural theory of mind, the 'super-ego':**
   A   Is unconscious.
   B   Contains values and moral rules.
   C   Conflicts with the 'id'.
   D   Always dictates behaviour consciously.
   E   Is the locus of repressed memories.

30.7   **The following statements are true of Freud's psychosexual stages of development:**
   A   Castration anxiety occurs in females during the genital stage.
   B   The anal stage is usually at age 3–5.
   C   The 'Oedipus complex' occurs during the 'oral' stage of development.
   D   The latency period is between the oral and anal stages.
   E   The 'Oedipus complex' refer to the male child's wish to kill the mother.

30.8   **The following statements about the post-Freudians are true.**
   A   Jung emphasised aggression rather then sex.
   B   Harry Stack-Sullivan coined the term 'organ inferiority'.
   C   Adler emphasised archetypes.
   D   Fromm-Reichmann emphasised interpersonal factors.
   E   Eric Erikson argued against a social perspective.

(Answers overleaf)

30.5 A **True**
B **False** This is the ego.
C **False**
D **True**
E **True**

(Further details can be found in the *Companion to Psychiatric Studies*, p. 850.)

30.6 A **False** It is partly conscious and partly unconscious.
B **True**
C **True**
D **False** Actions may be unconscious.
E **False**

(Further details can be found in the *Companion to Psychiatric Studies*, p. 850.)

30.7 A **False** It is a male child's response to fear of retaliation by his father during the Oedipus complex.
B **False** It is usually in the second year.
C **False** It occurs during the genital stage.
D **False** It is after the genital stage, at age 7 plus.
E **False** It refers to the child's wish to have an exclusive relationship with the mother and exclude or kill the father.

(Further details can be found in the *Companion to Psychiatric Studies*, p. 851.)

30.8 A **False** This was Adler.
B **False** This was Adler.
C **False** This was Jung.
D **True** Rather then Freudian intrapersonal emphasis.
E **False** He argued for it.

(Further details can be found in the *Companion to Psychiatric Studies*, pp. 851–852.)

30.9 **The following statements apply to the so-called object relations schools of analysis:**

A   Objects refers principally to the genitals.

B   The 'depressive position' occurs after the 'paranoid position'.

C   'Splitting' is a defence mechanism where good and bad objects cannot be integrated.

D   'Depressive anxiety' is the fear that one's love will destroy the object.

E   'Schizoid anxiety' is the fear that one's anger will destroy the object.

30.10 **Systematic desensitisation:**

A   Involves rapid exposure to a phobic object in a non-graded manner.

B   Was originally developed by Skinner in the 1940s.

C   Involves presenting phobic items in a hierarchical pattern.

D   Includes relaxation.

E   Involves only exposure 'in vivo'.

30.11 **Flooding:**

A   Is a form of systematic desensitisation.

B   Is a form of exposing patients to a phobic object in a graded manner.

C   Has relaxation to reduce anxiety as an important component.

D   Is usually is done in 10-minute sessions.

E   Is effective more rapidly than systematic desensitisation.

30.12 **The following are characteristics of standard cognitive therapy:**

A   The therapist adopts a passive accepting role.

B   The principal therapeutic method is Cartesian questioning.

C   It is closely related to rational–emotive therapy.

D   It emphasises the past history of the patient.

E   It is typically 30–50 sessions in duration.

(Answers overleaf)

30.9 A False Initially it is the mother's breast, then the whole person.
      B True Fear of being devoured is replaced by ambivalence.
      C True It is often described in 'borderline' personality disorder.
      D False This is schizoid anxiety.
      E False This is depressive anxiety.

(Further details can be found in the *Companion to Psychiatric Studies*, p. 852.)

30.10 A False It is gradual exposure – rapid is 'flooding'.
      B False It was developed by Wolpe in the 1950s.
      C True
      D True Relaxation inhibits anxiety.
      E False Imaginary exposure is also of established effectiveness.

(Further details can be found in the *Companion to Psychiatric Studies*, pp. 852–853.)

30.11 A False It involves rapid exposure.
      B False Presentation of objects is not graded.
      C False Relaxation is not typically included.
      D False Sessions are usually more than an hour long.
      E True But overall effectiveness is similar.

(Further details can be found in the *Companion to Psychiatric Studies*, p. 853.)

30.12 A False The therapist has an active and directive role throughout treatment.
      B False It is Socratic questioning.
      C True This was developed by Albert Ellis, who is credited with originating cognitive therapy together with Aaron Beck.
      D False It emphasises the 'here and now'.
      E False It is typically brief – 10–20 sessions.

(Further details can be found in the *Companion to Psychiatric Studies*, pp. 853–855.)

30.13   **The following individuals and concepts are related:**
   A   Jung and 'archetypes'.
   B   Beck and 'flooding'.
   C   Jung and 'individuation'.
   D   Erickson and 'basic trust versus mistrust'.
   E   Freud and 'splitting'.

30.14   **Elements of supportive psychotherapy include:**
   A   Reassurance.
   B   Ventilation.
   C   Behavioural modification.
   D   Analysis of transference.
   E   Guidance and suggestion.

(Answers overleaf)

30.13 A **True**
         B **False** Beck was an originator of cognitive therapy.
         C **True**
         D **True**
         E **False** This was Kline of the object relations school.

(Further details can be found in the *Companion to Psychiatric Studies*, pp. 850–854.)

30.14 A **True**
         B **True**
         C **False**
         D **False**
         E **True**

(Further details can be found in the *Companion to Psychiatric Studies*, p. 860.)

31. Evidence-based medicine and psychiatry

31.1 Evidence-based medicine (EBM):

A   Is concerned with treatment rather than diagnostic issues.

B   Depends upon precise formulation of an answerable clinical question.

C   Requires constant evaluation of one's clinical performance at each stage.

D   Involves the identification, critical appraisal and implementation of the best available evidence for a particular intervention in a given clinical situation.

E   Is an academic rather than a clinical pursuit.

31.2 Arguments for evidence-based medicine include:

A   Most clinical decisions made by doctors would change if the doctor had full access to all the available research evidence.

B   The further doctors are from graduation, the more out of date their practice becomes.

C   Continuing medical education does not work.

D   Textbooks are inevitably out of date by the time they are published.

E   Traditional review articles by self-professed experts are less systematic and more prone to bias than evidence-based reviews.

31.3 The Cochrane collaboration:

A   Was established to look at randomised controlled trials in general medicine.

B   Was established in 1982.

C   Incorporates five separate psychiatric review groups.

D   Only considers evidence from randomised controlled trials.

E   Established the Cochrane database of systematic reviews.

(Answers overleaf)

31.1 A **False** EBM equally applies to diagnosis, prognosis, etc.
      B **True**
      C **True**
      D **True**
      E **False** EBM is targeted at clinicians and doctors.

(Further details can be found in the *Companion to Psychiatric Studies*, p. 865.)

31.2 A **False** About 25% of decisions would change with greater access to evidence.
      B **True**
      C **True** Continuing medical education does not change clinical behaviour.
      D **True**
      E **True** There is a strong negative correlation between self-professed expertise and systematic reviewing.

(Further details can be found in the *Companion to Psychiatric Studies*, p. 866.)

31.3 A **False** Its remit includes all fields of medicine.
      B **False** It was established in 1992.
      C **True** They are schizophrenia, dementia, depression, drugs, developmental.
      D **False** Cochrane also registers trials in progress and high-quality reviews.
      E **True**

(Further details can be found in the *Companion to Psychiatric Studies*, pp. 866–867.)

31.4 **The following are components of the evidence-based medicine process:**

A   Framing answerable clinical questions.

B   Searching for evidence for and against a proposed intervention.

C   Appraising the evidence for and against a proposed intervention.

D   Adapting your clinical practice to incorporate the best evidence.

E   Evaluating your practice.

31.5 **The areas of practice covered by evidence-based medicine include:**

A   Treatment.

B   Diagnosis.

C   Clinical guidelines.

D   Health economics.

E   Aetiology.

31.6 **When framing a question prior to performing an evidence-based search:**

A   It is important that the question covers all the salient clinical details.

B   The question should have at least five parts.

C   The question should be expressed in numerical terms if possible.

D   The question should be tailored to the evidence with which you are already familiar.

E   Any given clinical scenario will generate a number of questions.

31.7 **When searching for evidence to answer a clinical question:**

A   A well-framed clinical question can make the literature search parameters obvious.

B   It is important not to change the question because the search is proving difficult.

C   It is best to limit the search to a small number of respected journals.

D   A search using an electronic database such as MEDLINE is likely to detect most of the relevant studies.

E   Searching the Cochrane library can be a useful short-cut.

(Answers overleaf)

31.4 A True
       B True
       C True
       D True
       E True

(Further details can be found in the *Companion to Psychiatric Studies*, p. 867.)

31.5 A True
       B True
       C True
       D True
       E True

(Further details can be found in the *Companion to Psychiatric Studies*, p. 867.)

31.6 A False All salient details would require several questions.
       B False It should have three or four parts.
       C False The question should be framed in 'search parameters'.
       D False This would bias the literature search.
       E True

(Further details can be found in the *Companion to Psychiatric Studies*, p. 868.)

31.7 A True
       B False It may be necessary to slightly modify the question.
       C False This would introduce bias.
       D False Only 30–50% of the relevant studies would be identified.
       E True It will identify relevant systematic reviews.

(Further details can be found in the *Companion to Psychiatric Studies*, p. 868.)

31.8   **When assessing whether the conclusions stated in a single treatment study are valid, the following are useful questions to ask:**
   A   Was the assignment of patients to treatment groups randomised?
   B   Was the randomisation list kept hidden from the researchers?
   C   Were the subjects blind to which treatment they were receiving?
   D   How many drop-outs were there?
   E   Were there any differences between the groups at the start of the trial?

31.9   **When critically appraising evidence from a treatment study:**
   A   A study may be scientifically valid without being clinically important.
   B   A study may be clinically important without being scientifically valid.
   C   The higher the NNT (number needed to treat), the more powerful the treatment effect.
   D   ARR (absolute risk reduction) is a measure of the difference in outcome between the different treatment groups in the study.
   E   NNT = 1/ARR.

31.10   **When incorporating research findings into your clinical practice:**
   A   It is important to ensure that your patient is similar to the subjects referred to in the papers that you are referencing.
   B   It should be possible to estimate whether your patient is likely to be more or less susceptible to the treatment than the average patient in the trial.
   C   As a practising clinician, you should not undertake an intervention unless there is sufficient research evidence to prove its effectiveness.
   D   It is important to go back and ask the same clinical question again.
   E   A critical professional culture will hinder the implementation of evidence-based medicine.

(Answers overleaf)

31.8   A   True
      B   True
      C   True
      D   True
      E   True

(Further details can be found in the *Companion to Psychiatric Studies*, p. 869 (Table 31.1).)

31.9   A   True
      B   False
      C   False   A lower NNT denotes a more powerful effect.
      D   True   It is sometimes denoted as CER–EER (control event rate–experimental event rate).
      E   True

(Further details can be found in the *Companion to Psychiatric Studies*, pp. 869–870.)

31.10   A   True
      B   True   It could be done by estimation or by reference to audit.
      C   False   Some interventions cannot be evaluated in RCTs.
      D   False   This is unnecessary.
      E   False   A supportive critical culture will foster EBM.

(Further details can be found in the *Companion to Psychiatric Studies*, p. 870.)

31.11   **With respect to current clinical practice:**
A   50% of all medical interventions are supported by solid scientific evidence.
B   Randomised controlled trials should be carried out to prove the efficacy of any established intervention for which there is no hard scientific evidence.
C   Individual case reports may identify effects that merit further study but are too susceptible to bias to be of general value.
D   There is more randomised controlled trial evidence for patient problems than for medical procedures.
E   Studies suggest that most patients admitted to acute general medical wards receive treatment that is evidence-based.

31.12   **With respect to current psychiatric practice:**
A   Studies suggest that most patients admitted to acute general psychiatric wards receive treatment that is evidence-based.
B   Studies suggest that the majority of psychiatric outpatients are not given treatments that are supported by randomised controlled trials.
C   The efficacy of antipsychotic medication in schizophrenia has been demonstrated in randomised controlled trials.
D   The efficacy of lithium augmentation therapy in treatment-resistant depression has been demonstrated in randomised controlled trials.
E   There is strong scientific evidence to support the use of constant nursing observation in patients at risk of suicide.

31.13   **Theoretical benefits of evidence-based medicine include:**
A   It helps new treatments to be incorporated into clinical practice earlier.
B   It helps reduce the number of ineffective interventions carried out.
C   It provides a common language and rules for communicating about effectiveness.
D   It improves undergraduate training and postgraduate education.
E   It increases clinical freedom.

(Answers overleaf)

31.11 A **False** Only about 15% of interventions are supported by evidence.
B **False** This may not be ethically possible.
C **True**
D **True** This is because common conditions are more likely to have been studied.
E **True** About 82% of these interventions are evidence-based.

(Further details can be found in the *Companion to Psychiatric Studies*, pp. 874–875.)

31.12 A **True** About 65% receive evidence-based treatment.
B **False** The majority get evidence-based treatment.
C **True**
D **True**
E **False**

(Further details can be found in the *Companion to Psychiatric Studies*, pp. 874–875.)

31.13 A **True**
B **True**
C **True**
D **True**
E **False**

(Further details can be found in the *Companion to Psychiatric Studies*, p. 876.)

Index

Abortions, therapeutic, 157
Abuse
   children, 181
   in psychiatric practice, 223
   sexual, 181
Academic psychiatry, 3
Adolescence disorders, 185–189
Adoption studies, 67
Advance directives, 229
Affective disorders *see* Mood disorders
Alcohol misuse/dependence, 97, 99
   adolescence, 187
   carry-over phenomenon, 101
   genetics, 99
   hallucinosis and, 101
   late-onset, 195
   prevention paradox, 95
   suicide and, 203
   women, 99
Alcohol use, regional differences, 95
Alzheimer's disease, 89
   cholinergic system, 15
   risk factors, 191
Amino acids, excitatory, 21
Amnesic syndrome, 9
Amygdala, 11
Anatomy *see* Neuroanatomy
Anorexia nervosa, 143, 145
   adolescence, 189
Anticholinergics, 39
Anticholinesterases, 23
Anticipation, 65
Antidepressants, 119
   new generation, 35
   overdoses, 35
   pharmacokinetics, 31, 33, 35
   pregnancy-related disorders, 159
   side-effects, 35
   tricyclic *see* Tricyclic antidepressants
   withdrawal syndromes, 37
Antipsychotics, 29, 31
Antisocial personality disorder, 167
Anxiety/Anxiety disorders, 77, 139
   adolescence, 185
   generalized anxiety disorder (GAD), 139
Arachnitis chronique, 3
Arousal response, 139

Arson, 219
Autism, 175, 177, 181
Automatism, 221
Avoidant personality disorder, 167

Basal ganglia, 5
Beneficence, 225
Benzodiazepines, 37, 39
Bipolar disorder, 113
   environmental risk factors, 115
Blood–brain barrier, 19
Borderline personality disorder, 167, 169
Brain
   energy and, 17
   functional neuroanatomy, 5
   imaging *see* Neuroimaging
   temporal lobe lesions, 89
Bulimia nervosa, 143, 145, 147
   adolescence, 189
Buspirone, 39

Cannabis, 101
Cell division, 59
Cerebellum, 5
Cerebral cortex, 5
Cerebrovascular accident, depression and, 91
Challenging behaviours, 177
Children
   abuse, 181
   development, 179, 181
   psychiatric disorders, 139, 179–184
Cholinergic neurotransmission, 23
Cholinergic system, 15
Chromosomes, 59
   DNA in, 61
Classification/Classification systems, 85, 87, 207
   early German, 3
Cochrane collaboration, 239
Cognitive development, 179
Cognitive therapy, 235
Compulsion, 229
Computerised tomography (CT), 129
Conduct disorder, 185
Confidentiality, 225, 227

Confounders, 57
Consciousness, mental state examination, 81
Consent, 227
Conversion disorder, 141, 211
Correlations, 47
Cotard's syndrome, 125
Creutzfeldt–Jakob disease (CJD), new variant, 89
Crime see Offenders

Defence mechanisms, 231
Delirium, 89, 191
Delusional disorders, 123, 125
Delusions, primary, 79
Dementia(s), 193
  causes, 89
  Down's syndrome, 173
  frontal, 7
  Lewy body, 191
  presenile, 89
  see also Alzheimer's disease
Depression
  adolescence, 189
  atypical, 111
  brief recurrent, 111
  characteristics, 79
  diagnostic criteria, 111
  genetic epidemiology, 113
  physical illness and, 207, 209
  post-stroke, 91
  postnatal, 159
  pregnancy, 157
  risk factors in women, 137
  suicide and, 201
  treatment, 119
Desensitisation, systematic, 235
Development
  cognitive, 179
  social, 181
Diagnosis, 85–88
DNA in chromosomes, 61
Doctor–patient relationship, 223
Dopamine, 25
Dopaminergic system, 11, 13
Dorsolateral prefrontal cortex (DLPFC) atrophy, 7
Down's syndrome, 173
Drinking behaviour, regional differences, 95
Drug misuse, 97
  mentally ill, 99
  prevention, 95
Drugs, 90

agonists/antagonists, 21
binding to receptors, 21, 133
biotransformation, 19
clearance, 19
pharmacokinetics, 17
routes of administration, 17
see also Pharmacology
DSM classification, 85
Dysmorphophobia, 125

Eating disorders, 143–148
  adolescence, 189
Ecological studies, 55
Elderly, 191–196
Electroconvulsive therapy (ECT), 119
Emotional disorders, childhood, 183
Encephalitis, herpes simplex, 9
Encopresis, 183
Endocrine system, neural regulation, 27
Enuresis, 183
Epidemiology, 51–58
  causes and mechanisms of diseases, 51
  measures in, 53, 55
Epilepsy, 91
Erectile dysfunction, 149, 151
Erection, 149, 151
Erotomania, 127
Ethics, 223–230
  research, 43
Evidence-based medicine, 239–246
Exhibitionism, 151

Factitious illness by proxy, 217
Family studies, 65
Fatigue, chronic, 211
Fetal alcohol syndrome, 101
Fitness to plead, 221
Flight of ideas, 77
Flooding, 235
Folie à deux, 127
Forensic psychiatry, 215–222
Fragile X syndrome, 175
Freud, Sigmund, 233

GABA receptors, 21
Ganglion cells, retinal, 5
Ganser syndrome, 127
Generalized anxiety disorder (GAD), 139
Genes, linkage analysis, 69, 71
Genetics, 59–72

Hallucinosis, alcoholic, 101
Heroin addiction, 97
Herpes simplex encephalitis, 9
Hippocampus, 9
  schizophrenia, 9, 11
Hippocratic Oath, 223, 225
History, 1–4
Homosexuality, 151
Hospital orders, 221
Huntington's disease (chorea), 7, 93
Hydrocephalus, normal pressure, 93
Hyperemesis gravidarum, 157
Hyperkinetic disorder, 183
Hypochondriacal psychosis (delusions),
    monosymptomatic, 125
Hypochondriasis, 211
Hypothalamus, 11

ICD-10, 85
'Id', 233
Imprinting, 65
Indecent exposure, 151, 219
Infanticide, 221
Inheritance/Inherited disorders, 61, 63
  learning disability, 175
Interviewing, 73–76

Jealousy, morbid, 125

Klinefelter's syndrome, 173
Klüver–Bucy syndrome, 9
Kraepelin, Emil, 3

Laing, R.D., 225
Law/Legal issues
  history, 1
  mentally disordered offenders, 219,
    221
Learning disability, 171–178
  criminal behaviour and, 217
Lewy body dementia, 191
Liaison psychiatry, 205–214
Limbic system, 7
Lithium, adverse effects/toxicity, 37

Magnetic resonance imaging (MRI), 129
  functional, 129, 131
Magnetic resonance spectroscopy
    (MRS), 129, 131
Mania, 111, 121

Marijuana, 101
Maternity blues, 159
Memory
  loss, 9
  neurobiology, 9, 11
  short-term, 81
Menopause, 155
Mental state examination, 77–84
Meta-analysis, 49
Monoamine oxidase inhibitors (MAOIs),
  33
Mood, elevated, 79
Mood disorders, 111–122
  elderly, 193
  environmental risk factors, 115
  sleep disturbance, 117
  treatment, 119, 121
Movement disorders, schizophrenia, 77
Multiple sclerosis, 93

Naming, disorder of, 83
National Psychiatric Morbidity
    Household Survey (NPMS),
    137
Neuroanatomy, functional, 5–16
Neuroimaging, 129–130
  drug binding studies, 133
  functional, 129, 131, 133
  quantitative scan analysis, 133
Neuroleptics see Antipsychotics
Neuronal signalling, 19
Neurones, dopaminergic, 11
Neuropharmacology, 17–28
Neuroses, 137–142
  childhood, 139
  outcome factors, 137
Neurotransmission, 23
Nicotinic receptor antagonists, 23
Non-maleficence, 225
Noradrenaline, 25
Noradrenergic neurotransmission, 23
Noradrenergic system, 13

Obsessive–compulsive disorder, 141
  adolescence, 185
Offenders
  genetic factors, 215
  intelligence, 215
  mentally disordered, 217, 219, 221
  recidivism, 217
  sexual, 153
Old age psychiatry, 191–196
Opioid drugs, 27

Organic disorders, 89–94
Othello syndrome, 125

Panic disorder, 209
Paranoid disorders, 123–128
Parkinson's disease, 25
Penile erection, 149, 151
Perception abnormalities, 81
Personality/Personality theories, 163–165
Personality disorders, 165–170
Pharmacokinetics, 17
Pharmacology
    neuropharmacology, 17–28
    psychopharmacology, 29–40
Phenothiazines, 31
Phobias, social, 141
Physical illness, psychiatric disorders
        and, 205, 207, 209
Pinel, Philippe, 1, 3
Population attributable fraction, 55
Postconcussional syndrome, 91
Postnatal depression, 159
Postpartum psychosis, 159, 161
Post-traumatic stress disorder, 141
Prefrontal circuit, 7
Pregnancy, 157
    depression, 157
    teenage, 187
Premenstrual syndrome (PMS), 155
Pseudodementia, depressive, 195
Psychopharmacology, 29–40
Psychosis
    functional, elderly, 193
    postpartum, 159, 161
Psychotherapy, 231–238
    supportive, 231, 232

Randomized controlled trials, 57
Rating scales, 45
Recombination, genetics, 71
Research, 41–50
    data, 43
    epidemiology, 55, 57
    ethics, 43
    statistics in, 45, 47
    study design, 41, 55

Schizoid personality disorder, 167
Schizophrenia, 103–110
    adolescence, 189
    aetiology, 107
    epidemiology, 105

'first-rank' symptoms, 79
    hippocampus in, 9, 11
    hypofrontality in, 7
    learning disability and, 177
    movement disorders, 77
    outcome, 109
    phenomenology, 103
    psychological theories, 107
    suicide and, 201
    symptoms, 79, 105
    thought disorder in, 77, 105
    treatment, 109
    varieties and related conditions, 105
Schizotypal personality disorder, 167
School refusal, 183
Seasonal affective disorder (SAD), 113
Seizures, 91
Self-harm, deliberate, 203
    adolescents, 189
    biological variables, 199
    elderly, 195
Senile squalor, 195
Sensory systems, 5
Serotonergic system, 13, 15
Serotonin receptors, 27
Serotonin reuptake inhibitors, 27, 35, 119
Sex therapy, 149
Sexual disorders, 149–154
    drug treatment, 151
Sexual offenders, 153
Sexual orientation, 151
Shell shock, 3
Sidaway case, 227
Single photon emission tomography
        (SPECT), 131
Sleep disturbance, mood disorders,
        117
Social development, 181
Social phobia, 141
Soiling, 183
Somatic symptoms, 205
Somatisation disorder, 141, 209
Somatoform disorder, 205
Standard deviation (SD), 45
Starvation, metabolic consequences,
        147
Statistical parametric mapping (SPM),
        135
Statistical power, 57
Statistical tests, 47
Statistics, 45, 47
Stroke, depression and, 91
Stupor, psychogenic, 83
Substance misuse, 95–102
    adolescence, 187

medical patients, 213
see also Alcohol misuse/dependence;
  Drug misuse
Suicide, 197–201
  adolescents, 189
  elderly, 195
  mental illness and, 201
  methods, 197
  rates, 197
  young males, 199
'Super-ego', 233
Survival analysis, 47
Symptoms, 'first-rank', 81
  schizophrenia, 79
Szasz, Thomas, 225

Tarasoff Judgement, 227
Temporal lobe lesions, 89
Thought disorder in schizophrenia, 77,
  105

Trait personality theory, 163
Transcranial magnetic stimulation
  (TMS), 135
Transference, 231
Transsexualism, 153
Tricyclic antidepressants, 31, 33
Tryptophan depletion, 117
Tuberose sclerosis, 175
Twin studies, 67, 69

Violent patients, interviewing, 73

Wernicke–Korsakoff syndrome, 9, 91
Women's disorders, 155–162
World War I, 3

X-linked disorders, 63
X-ray computerised tomography, 129